T0219738

Ihr Bonus als Käufer dieses Buches

Als Käufer dieses Buches können Sie kostenlos unsere Flashcard-App „SN Flashcards"
mit Fragen zur Wissensüberprüfung und zum Lernen von Buchinhalten nutzen.
Für die Nutzung folgen Sie bitte den folgenden Anweisungen:

1. Gehen Sie auf **https://flashcards.springernature.com/login**
2. Erstellen Sie ein Benutzerkonto, indem Sie Ihre Mailadresse angeben,
   ein Passwort vergeben und den Coupon-Code einfügen.

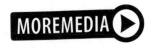

Ihr persönlicher „SN Flashcards"-App Code   24EF5-54A83-EEA13-B5953-63EB2

Sollte der Code fehlen oder nicht funktionieren, senden Sie uns bitte eine E-Mail mit
dem Betreff **„SN Flashcards"** und dem Buchtitel an **customerservice@springernature.com**.

Fachenglisch für BioTAs und BTAs

Ursula Steiner

Fachenglisch für BioTAs und BTAs

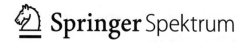

Ursula Steiner
Isny im Allgäu, Deutschland

ISBN 978-3-662-60665-0   ISBN 978-3-662-60666-7 (eBook)
https://doi.org/10.1007/978-3-662-60666-7

Die Deutsche Nationalbibliothek verzeichnet diese Publikation in der Deutschen Nationalbibliografie; detaillierte bibliografische Daten sind im Internet über http://dnb.d-nb.de abrufbar.

Springer Spektrum
© Springer-Verlag GmbH Deutschland, ein Teil von Springer Nature 2020, korrigierte Publikation 2020

Planung/Lektorat: Stephanie Preuß
Springer Spektrum ist ein Imprint der eingetragenen Gesellschaft Springer-Verlag GmbH, DE und ist ein Teil von Springer Nature.
Die Anschrift der Gesellschaft ist: Heidelberger Platz 3, 14197 Berlin, Germany

I dedicate this book to
Prof. Dr. Gerald Grübler
who has always supported me regarding
international relationships.

Educational Objectives

Aim of this book is to broaden your horizon about:

▶ **Technical knowledge:** To give an insight of a great spectrum of biotechnology and thus leading to an enrichment of biotechnological vocabulary.

▶ **Methodological knowledge**: Knowledge about how to analyse specific texts and how to revise vocabulary in a versatile way.

▶ **Social competence:** Exchange ideas and further knowledge with your partner. Being able to express your opinion and form a statement with sophisticated arguments.

▶ **Interdisciplinary competence:** Teachers of biotechnology and chemistry as well as English teachers should work together and set into practice teamteaching to give an example for the best result of interdisciplinary work and to encourage pupils to look for an interdisciplinary scientific approach which is tremendously important for the innovation in biotechnology. Exercises which can be done in teamteaching are marked with *.

Acknowledgements

I thank Prof. Dr. h.c. Wagner for sustaining me to promote the book. I explicitly thank Prof. Dr. Heiner Quast for his extraordinary valuable advice and I also would like to thank Dr. Preuss, Mr. Thachancheri, Mrs. Schänfler and Mrs. Krieger for the vivid creation of the book. Most of all I thank all authors, editors, scientists and companies that were so kindly to give me the permission to print their work for educational purposes. In addition I thank Mr. Lay for his technical support and the PTAs for the listening comprehension.

Introduction to the Book

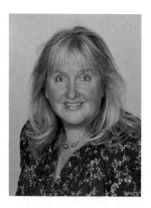

This textbook was arranged in accordance with the curriculum of the federal state Baden-Württemberg by Ursula Steiner. Baden-Württemberg is the only federal state which has established the education biotechnological assistant. As there is no book available on the market for BIOTAs she thought it would finally be a good idea to gather all her 16 years teaching experience into a book.

Mrs. Steiner is teaching English, specific English at the vocational college for biotechnological assistants, chemical technical assistants, pharmaceutical technical assistants, assistants in physics and assistants in information and communication technology. Beyond that she gives lectures in Business English and technical English at the University of Applied Sciences for chemists, information technologists and physicists.

Furthermore she is teaching economics and social studies. She is head of the international office.

In addition she documented and coordinated a BMBF (Bundesministerium für Bildung und Forschung = Ministry for Education and Research) project about vocational education in China and established the children's university with Prof. Dr. Axel Hoff.

It would be a pleasure for her if this book is a help for BIOTAs as nowadays English is indispensible in sciences.

In 2018 a turnover of 4,150 billion euro was generated by 646 biotechnological companies in Germany with 21.860 employees. 50.5 % of biotechnological companies work in the field of health and medicine (source: www.biotechnologie.de).

Table of Contents

Biotechnology

1

Contents

Introduction to Red Biotechnology

Biotechnology derives from the Greek words – bios – life, technos – technology and logos – language, proof – that is biotechnology deals with the technical usage of living organisms for various purposes such as food, medicine, pharmaceuticals, recycling. Nowadays we deal with various colours or categories namely 10 introduced (red, blue, green, white, grey, yellow, brown, violet, dark and gold biotechnology) by Dr. Rita R. Colwell in 2003 and presented in this book. Other categories are also in use, the division into plant

Die Originalversion dieses Kapitels wurde korrigiert. Ein Erratum finden Sie unter
https://doi.org/10.1007/978-3-662-60666-7_13

© Springer-Verlag GmbH Deutschland, ein Teil von Springer Nature 2020
U. Steiner, *Fachenglisch für BioTAs und BTAs*,
https://doi.org/10.1007/978-3-662-60666-7_1

Tab. 1.1 Vocabulary for
the introduction to red
biotechnology

English	German
genetic engineering	Gentechnik
genetic makeup	genetischer Aufbau
vaccines	Impfstoffe
tissue engineering	Gewebetechnik
cartilage	Knorpel
disc replacement	Bandscheibenersatz
amplifications	Vervielfältigungen
genetic disposition	genetische Veranlagung

biotechnology, animal biotechnology, biotechnology of microorganisms and its colonies, cell culture biotechnologies, biotechnology of subcellular systems. The word 'biotechnology' was used for the first time by the director of the cattle utilization cooperative and Hungarian great land owner Karl Ereky and latter Hungarian Food minister (source:www.101jahre-biotech.de). He published a book with the title: "Biotechnology of the meat, fat and milk production in agricultural large concerns for scientific sophisticated farmers" in 1919 in Berlin. His idea was to produce consumer goods with the use of living organisms called biotechnology. That was nothing new, but the word was new.

So lets immerse in the world of biotechnology which is as colourful and fascinating as life itself.

Red biotechnology deals with biotechnological techniques such as gene therapy (replacing a defective gene causing diseases by a healthy gene), stem cell research (to fight off leukaemia), **genetic engineering** (changing the **genetic makeup** of genes to produce improved organisms) and the development of new drugs and **vaccines** in medicine.

Another inventive application is **tissue engineering**. That means that cells are cultivated for tissue implantation. This leads to the production of artificial skin, **cartilage** and spinal **disc replacement**.

Furthermore red biotechnology finds also its application in the field of research about mutations and **amplifications** of genes to cure degenerative diseases such as Parkinson.

It is commonly known that certain drugs are not so effective for every patient because of its **genetic disposition** and metabolism. Therefore knowing the genetic disposition of a patient implies a better treatment by the analysis of the genes.

In conclusion red biotechnology means an immense progress in medicine which still has to be developed further.

Tab. 1.2 Vocabulary for the text red biotechnology: Parkinson's disease: vitamin B3 has a positive effect on nerve cells

English	German
impairment	Verschlechterung
to boost	ankurbeln
to come up with	darauf kommen
hence	daher
the sought after component	gefragte Komponente
the latter	Letzteres
the precursor	Vorläufer
the elevation	Herausnahme
adverse effects	Gegenauswirkungen
phytochemicals	sekundärer Pflanzenstoff (Chemikalien, die in Pflanzen vorkommen)

1.1   Red Biotechnology (Tab. 1.2)

Parkinson's Disease: Vitamin B3 Has a Positive Effect on Nerve Cells

Parkinson's disease is one of the most common neurodegenerative diseases in the world. There are around 4.1 million sufferers worldwide. It is characterised by motor **impairments** that result from the death of certain nerve cells in the brain. Therapies are not yet available. However, researchers at the University of Tübingen have now discovered that vitamin B3 has a positive effect on damaged nerve cells and can **boost** their energy metabolism. Vitamin B3 application will now be examined to determine whether it could be a new therapeutic approach for treating Parkinson's.

Parkinson's is the second most common neurodegenerative disease after Alzheimer's. The disease affects around two percent of people over 60 worldwide, and the numbers are rising. Between 250,000 and 280,000 people have the disease in Germany alone. Typical symptoms of this still incurable disease include motor impairments such as unsteady hands, stiff muscles and slow movements. The disease is caused by the loss of dopamine-containing nerve cells in a certain brain region called the black substance (substantia nigra). Little is yet known why these nerve cells die.

For many years, junior professor Dr. Dr. Michela Deleidi and her research group at the Hertie Institute for Clinical Brain Research and the University of Tübingen have been studying how Parkinson's disease develops. "Some time ago, we **came up with** the idea that the disease is caused by damaged nerve cells with a dysfunctional energy metabolism, and **hence** damaged mitochondria," explains Deleidi. "And indeed, in one of our studies, we found that the mitochondria in the affected nerve cells of Parkinson's patients did not work properly. So we then decided to look for a way to repair and improve mitochondrial function."

In search of a "mitochondrial rescue", as Deleidi calls it, the researchers came across vitamin B3. "It has long been known that vitamin B3 plays a role in central metabolic processes, and some studies have shown that the vitamin plays a role in maintaining healthy mitochondria," says the neurologist. "So it was natural for us to look at the vitamin and its potential role in the treatment of Parkinson's."

Vitamin B3 Can Save Nerve Cells

The scientists took skin cell samples from patients with Parkinson's, i.e. patients that carried a defect in the so-called GBA *gene, in order to find out whether damaged mitochondria cause Parkinson's disease. A mutation in this gene is one of the major risk factors for Parkinson's disease. After removal, the cells were converted into stem cells using protocols that were developed specifically for this purpose. "All artificial nerve cells had a characteristic mutation in the GBA gene, which is the most frequent risk gene for Parkinson's," says Deleidi "And we were able to show that the mitochondria and energy metabolism of these cells were impaired."

The scientists from Tübingen subsequently treated the damaged cells with a vitamin B3 variant. "And fortunately, we were able to eliminate most of the cells' abnormalities," said the junior professor. "In the flies that we were using as models of ageing, we even found that **the sought after compound** is a true anti-ageing product." The researchers, who are part of an international research consortium, took flies of the genus *Drosophila* that had a defective GBA gene and hence problems moving around, and fed them the vitamin B3 variant to boost the formation of new mitochondria. "And there too, we were able to show that the vitamin considerably improved neuronal functions and behaviour," says Deleidi.

Nicotinamide Riboside Improves Cellular Energy Production

The researchers did not use vitamin B3 – the nicotinamide – for the investigations, but a variant of the vitamin called nicotinamide riboside. **The latter** is **the precursor** of the coenzyme NAD (nicotinamide adenine dinucleotide), which plays an important role in many metabolic processes involved cellular energy production. "We now know that the administration of the vitamin B3 variant nictoinamide riboside leads to **the elevation** of the intracellular NAD level and hence to considerable improvement of many biological processes, including microchondrial function and cellular energy generation," said the researcher. "Our experiments suggest that the loss of mitochondria does indeed play a significant role in the development of Parkinson's disease."

Vitamin B3 – A Universal Anti-Ageing Product?

Administering nicotinamide riboside may be a new starting point for treating Parkinson's. "At present, several clinical trials involving healthy volunteers and people with other mitochondrial diseases are underway." "The goal is to find out how the vitamin B3 variant works", says Deleidi. "While we are waiting for these results to be available we will continue characterising the substance and its metabolism in greater detail. Previous studies indicate that the vitamin B3 variant does not lead to serious **adverse effects**. However, the dosage will have to be very high because the drug needs to be taken orally. I am often asked by patients if they can start taking the substance. But I think that we need more results before giving the go-ahead for this."

The researchers are already working with ChromaDex on the optimisation of nicotinamide riboside. ChromaDex is an American company that specialises in **phytochemicals** and has already supplied the Tübingen researchers with nicotinamide riboside for a recently completed study. "In addition to our previous findings, the study shows that our approach is not only specifically directed at the age-related degradation of metabolic processes in the human body, which includes Alzheimer's, muscle loss and eye problems," says Deleidi. And the sooner you can do something about this, the better. If the outcome of the clinical trials is positive, vitamin B3 would really have what it takes to become the new "anti-ageing pill".

*GBA = Genombezeichnung

1.1.1   General Questions

1. First of all write a summary of the text. Use your own words.
2. Research the following terms with your partner. State your sources. Find five facts about:*
   a) Vitamin B3
   b) Nicotinamide riboside
   c) Parkinson's disease
   d) Mitochondria
   e) GBA gene
   f) metabolism
3. Explain the causes of Parkinson's disease!
4. Describe how the researchers found out that vitamin B3 has a positive effect on damaged nerve cells?
5. Outweigh the chances about curing Parkinson according to this research. Name two pros and two cons and draw a conclusion.
6. Complete the sentences:

Red biotechnology means to me…
Alzheimer's and Parkinson's disease…
Vitamin B 3…

7. Find the synonyms and antonyms:

synonyms	antonyms
goal	impairment
to boost	precursor
around	degradation

1.1.2   Vocabulary

Complete the table:

Noun	Verb	Adjective
	to involve	
		adverse
degradation		
		metabolic
removal		

Make up a sentence with four words of the table:

e.g. Many researchers were involved in this project.

1.1.3   Grammar

State the name of the tenses, give reasons why they were used:

1. Researchers at the University of Tübingen **have** now **discovered** that vitamin B 3 **has** a positive effect on damaged nerve cells.
2. For many years researchers **have been studying** how Parkinson's disease develops.
3. While **we are waiting** for these results, to be available, we will continue characterising the substance and its metabolism in greater detail.

1.1.4 Vocabulary

Find the words in English: the numbers of the letters form a new word:
e.g. removal:

richtig	–	right	–	1st letter
entfernen	–	eliminate	–	1st letter
machen	–	make	–	1st letter
Wahl	–	option	–	1st letter
bewegen	–	move	–	3rd letter
Anwendung	–	application	–	1st letter
Ziel	–	goal	–	4th letter

Now it is your turn:

ansteigen	_____	-	1st letter
Leidtragende	_____	-	5th letter
beträchtlich	_____	-	6th letter
erhältlich	_____	-	7th letter
Verschlechterung	_____	-	1st letter
Ergebnis	_____	-	1st letter
Anwendung	_____	-	8th letter
regulieren	_____	-	8th letter
umwandeln	_____	-	1st letter
Forscher	_____	-	8th letter
unheilbar	_____	-	2nd letter
Entnahme	_____	-	4th letter
löschen	_____	-	3rd letter
Anstrengung	_____	-	4th letter
Alterung	_____	-	2nd letter
hintereinander folgend	_____	-	12th letter (adverb)

1.1.5   Draw a Mindmap About

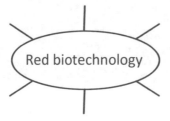

1.1.6   Translation

See Figs. 1.1 and 1.2

Tandem partner A

Partner A translates text A. Partner B has the solution and corrects it.

1. Rote Biotechnologie wird für die medizinische Diagnostik verwendet.

2. Es ist seit langem bekannt, dass Vitamin B3 bei metabolischen Prozessen eine große Rolle spielt.

3. Die Bewegungsabläufe werden durch Parkinson verschlechtert.

4. Die Funktion und das Verhalten von Neuronen werden durch Vitamin B3 verbessert.

Partner B translates text B. Partner A has the solution and corrects it.

1. There has been no therapy so far against Parkinson's.

2. The mutation of the GBA gene is the main risk factor for Parkinson's.

3. The scientists are already working on an optimisation of the therapy.

4. The scientific approach is not only directed for Parkinson's, but also for all other diseases.

Fig. 1.1 Tandem partner A

Tandem partner B

Partner B translates text B. Partner A has the solution and corrects it.

1. Bis jetzt gibt es noch keine Therapie gegen Parkinson.

2. Die Mutation des GBA Gens ist der hauptsächliche Risikofaktor für Parkinson.

3. Die Wissenschaftler arbeiten schon an einer Optimierung der Therapie.

4. Der wissenschaftliche Ansatz ist nicht nur auf Parkinson ausgerichtet, sondern auch für alle anderen altersbedingten Krankheiten relevant.

Partner A translates text A. Partner B has the solution and corrects it.

1. Red biotechnology is used for the medical diagnostics.

2. It has been known for a long time, that vitamin B3 plays an important role in metabolic processes.

3. The course of motions is getting impaired by Parkinson's.

4. The function and the behaviour of neurones are improved by vitamin B3.

Fig. 1.2 Tandem partner B

1.1.7   Definitions

Find the definitions for the following words or find the words for the definitions:

_____ - the modification of genes to cure illnesses

_____ - tests to prove the efficiency of a pharmaceutical drug

_____ - if the health condition of a person gets worse

Phytochemicals - _____

Neurodegenerative disease -_____

Substantia nigra - _____

1.1.8   Important Words in the Field of Red Biotechnology

Nouns	Verbs	Adjectives
alleviation – Linderung	to enhance the quality of life – die Lebensqualität verbessern	acellular – zelllos
agent – Wirkstoff	to administer sth. – etw. regeln	incurable – unheilbar
antibiotics – Antibiotika	to impair – sich verschlechtern	metabolic – metabolisch
biopharmaceuticals – Biopharmazeutika	to transcribe – übertragen	mitochondrial – mitochondrial
diagnostics – Diagnostik	to validate – etw. für gültig erklären	carcinogen – krebserregend
genetic engineering – Gentechnologie	to modify – verändern	homologous – ursprungsgleich
intellectual property – geistiges Eigentum	to come across sth. – auf etw stoßen	in vivo – im lebenden Organismus
tissue engineering – Gewebetechnologie	to convert into sth. – in etw umwandeln	adaptive – angepasst
vaccine – Impfstoff	to amplify – vervielfältigen	intercalated – eingefügt
clinical trial – klinischer Versuch	to invaginate – einstülpen	additive – hinzugefügt

1.2   Blue Biotechnology

Introduction to Blue Biotechnology
Blue biotechnology deals with aquatic organisms. These organisms are used for pharmaceutical drugs, cosmetics or research. E.g. algae can be used for food, drugs and biofuels. **Jellyfish** can be used for research of neurons by exploiting their fluorescence. The government of Bill Clinton set a huge amount of money free to do research in this field as there is still a lot of unknown sealife in the ocean. Most of our world is covered with water. Without water there is no life.

Vocabulary: jellyfish – Qualle

Watch the YouTube video:

Marine biotechnology: www.youtube.com/watch?v=hv1U19J3yfw

Name 5 marine organisms which appeared in the video.

1.2.1   General Text (Tab. 1.3)

Tab. 1.3 Vocabulary for the text Marine biotechnology: unknown sources of hope from depths of the sea

English	German
to revolve around	kursieren
bandied around	Gerüchte verbreiten
to come in	mit sich bringen
sponges	Schwämme
anti-inflammatory	entzündungshemmend
at random	zufällig
soy	Soja
rapeseed	Raps
washing detergents	wäschmittel
sessile animals	festgewachsene Organismen
predators	Raubtiere
scare off	abschrecken
habitat	Lebensraum
commodities	Wirtschaftsgüter
metabolite	Stoffwechselprodukt
ex situ	Maßnahmen, die außerhalb des eigentlichen Lebensraums stattfinden
brominated	bromiert
scarce	selten
to clamour	lautstark fordern
to trigger	auslösen

Unknown Sources of Hope from Depths of the Sea

Green, red, white and blue – the colours of biotechnology. Blue, i.e. marine biotechnology, is one of the less known branches. Biotechnological methods are used to
investigate marine life and the results obtained from these investigations advance
research in the fields of medicine and energy and into substances used as food supplements and cosmetics. The area of marine biotechnology is fairly diverse. Although it is not on the coast, even the southern German state of Baden-Württemberg
is involved in marine biotechnology.

The sea – the yrr∗ invented by German science fiction author Frank Schätzing
live in it, Jules Verne's protagonists travel 20,000 leagues under it and SpongeBob's
pineapple house sits on its bed. Only around one percent of the ocean has been stu-
died, which is why a lot of myths, speculation and fairytales **revolve around** it.
However, new terms like "drugstore from the bottom of the sea" or "marine pharmacy" have started to be **bandied around**. Marine microorganisms have had around
three billion years more to develop than life on land. They have adapted to extreme
environmental conditions in the sea – from the cold of the Antarctic ice to the hot,
bubbling deep-sea volcanoes. This is where biotechnology **comes in**, or rather marine biotechnology, to be more exact. Marine biotechnology is the application of
science and technology to marine organisms. Marine microbes, **sponges** and algae
produce substances that have been found to be effective against cancer and AIDS,
they are also likely to become important **providers** of energy, they are used to produce substances such as glass or to obtain important knowledge for the production
of new **washing detergents** active at lower temperatures.

Some pharmaceutical substances isolated from marine organisms have already
been placed on the market. Rather like tiny factories embedded in coral reefs, cyanobacteria, also known as blue algae, are among the most important producers of a
broad range of different substances (more than 200), including bioactive with anti-
tumour, antibiotic, **anti-inflammatory** and antiviral effect.

Yrr∗ – fictious, marine, unicellular jelly-like life form whose mission is to eliminate the human race by devasting the Earth's oceans. The protagonist of the novel,
Norwegian scientist Sigur Johanson, calls this life form "yrr", a name he created by
typing three letters **at random** on his keyboard (eds. note).

Biotechnological Research Involving Marine Organisms

Algae have the potential to be used in many different areas. They produce hydrogen, which will make them important sources of energy in the future; algae genes
are transferred into **soy** and **rapeseed**, where they lead to the increased production
of omega-3 fatty acids, essential fatty acids that cannot be synthesised by the human
body, but are vital for normal metabolism. Researchers also focus on marine sponges, small **sessile animals** that have colonised the oceans for around 800 million
years and developed an arsenal of mechanisms to defend themselves against **predators**.

The substances, which **scare** predators **off** rather than killing them, contain toxic and pharmaceutically active substances which are now used in cancer research, in particular in leukaemia research.

Only a small fraction of biotechnological research – around one percent – involves marine organisms. Marine research is very expensive and the prospect of commericialising new discoveries is still a distant dream. The coastal states of Bremen and Schleswig-Holstein are leaders in the field of marine biotechnology in Germany. The Helmholtz Centre for Ocean Research in Kiel – GEOMAR – investigates the chemical, physical, biological and geological processes of all marine **habitats** and is also active in the field of marine microbiology. "Many of our projects are focused on marine microorganisms from which we can isolate natural substances. We are also very much focused on turning our research results into marketable **commodities**," said Johanna Silber of GEOMAR, going to add that GEOMAR has already identified a number of marine microbial compounds that are used in cosmetics, antibiotics and even pesticides.

Sessile Organisms as Pharmaceutical Factories

Despite the fact that Baden-Württemberg is not on the coast, the marine life sciences branch is nevertheless represented here in the form of sponge and algae projects. Even a sponge species was discovered in Baden Württemberg: *Tethya wilhelma* was discovered and characterised by Franz Brümmer and Dr. Michael Nickel in the zoo "Wilhelma" (Stuttgart) around ten years ago. The small, white sponge is ball-shaped. But what differentiates it from all other sponge species is that it is able to move around.

Researchers at the Karlsruhe Institute of Technology are focused on marine sponges and algae. Using *Aplysina aerophoba*, also known as Gold-sponge, as a model organism, Christoph Syldatk and his team are studying the **metabolite** production of **ex situ** sponge cultures. They are particularly interested in improving the cultivation of sponges from a biotechnological point of view. Cultivating sponges with the aim of producing bioactive substances in relatively large quantities has always been very difficult.

Aplysina aerophoba is a common sponge in the Mediterranean. It is of great interest to researchers due to its ability to produce the pharmaceutically active substance aeroplysinin-1 as a natural metabolite. The **brominated** low-molecular metabolite has an antibacterial effect and also impairs the growth of tumor cells. Although aeroplysinin-1 is commercially available, it still needs to be extracted from sponges. Sponge-associated microorganisms have also been found to produce some of the bioactive natural substances that were previously thought to have been produced by the sponge.

Algal Bioreactors from Baden-Württemberg with Great Potential for the Future

The energy sector is another important area of application for marine biotechnology. When energy is **scarce**, people tend to **clamour** for new, efficient and environmentally friendly energy carriers. In addition, new energy sources must have an environmentally friendly CO_2 balance and must not use land set aside for agriculture. Algae could be a way out of this situation. Algae are relatively versatile; they can be used as food supplements and to produce biodiesel, oil and bioethanol. In addition, algal bioreactors like the ones produced by Baden-Württemberg-based Subitec GmbH can be set up anywhere. Subitec optimises its bioreactors for the cultivation of marine and freshwater algae according to the specific requirements of its clients. Many products can be produced with algae, including substances used as food supplements or in the cosmetics industry. Dr. Peter Ripplinger, CEO of Susitec, also points out that raw materials such as carbohydrates and lipids could be produced with algae as energy producers." Future energy production will not be dominated by rapeseed; I firmly believe that the future production of energy from biomass will be based on algae", said Ripplinger.

Algae bind CO_2 as they grow. However, this CO_2 is released when energy is produced. Algae can therefore be characterised as CO_2 neutral. However, they can do even better than that: Prof. Clemen Posten and his team at the Karlsruhe Institute of Technology are working on bioprocesses that enable them to cultivate the green alga *Chlamydomonas reinhardtii* in a way that **triggers** it to produce environmentally-friendly hydrogen, both more cheaply and more energy efficiently than has been possible up until now.

Processing of Marine Waste in Europe

Marine waste can be further processed using biotechnological methods. Chitin, which is found in the shells of shellfish that are removed prior to being packed and sold – quantities of around 750,000 t of shells per year are removed in Europe – is already being converted into chitosan in Asia. Chitosan is still very much in its infancy in Europe. The shells of European shellfish contain too much chalk which renders the further processing of chitin into chitosan uneconomical. However, the "ChiBo" project, which is funded under the European 7th Framework Programme, is seeking to improve the situation.

The Fraunhofer Institute for Interfacial Engineering and Biotechnology (IGB) in Stuttgart is part of the project and is focused on the development of enzymes that degrade chitin into monomers. Dr. Antje Laber (GEOMAR) does not regard marine biotechnology as a different branch of traditional biotechnology. "We are working with the same methods, devices and principles as the other branches. The only difference is that we are working with algae. I imagine that the potential of new characteristics and potentials offered by marine substances will in future become an integral part of classical biotechnology," Laber said. And what this means in concrete terms is that marine biotechnology can support and stimulate the other branches of biotechnology with its findings.

1.2.2   General Questions

1. State at least two advantages and disadvantages of blue biotechnology. Draw a conclusion!
2. Explain the advantages of algae in comparison to other fuels.
3. Name at least one application of blue biotechnology* in the field of:
   a) research
   b) medicine
   c) pharmaceutical use
   d) waste recycling
   e) cosmetics
Complete your answers by doing research in the internet. State your sources!*
4. Find out five facts about GEOMAR!
5. Give a closer definition of chitin!*

1.2.3   Description

Find five facts about these marine organisms in the field of biotechnology:*
   cyanobacteria

   sponges

   algae

1.2.4   Categories

Find at least for three categories examples of marine life.*
   Write three examples for each category!

Category 1: molluscs – Weichtiere	Category 2: invertebrates – wirbellose Tiere	Category 3: marine microorganisms – Meeresmikroorganismen

Find out which relationship they have with blue biotechnology. E.g. can they be used as pharmaceuticals for medical research or as biofuel?

1.2.5   Grammar

Find 5 adjectives in the text:	Find 5 adverbs in the text:

1. Make up a sample sentence with each.
2. Describe one biotechnological tool, biotechnological product or a biotechnological marine organism with at least 5 adjectives or 5 adverbs.

1.2.6   Vocabulary

Scrambled words: Put the letters into the right order

pssgnoe	
esselis	
sprdarote	
ticaaqu	
rasetbetrev	

1.2.7   Matching Sentences Together

Put the sentences into the right order

1. temperature – light - vary on – habitats – currents – salinity.
2. the shore - live – most - to – invertebrates – close – marine.
3. float - to swim - not – able – plankton – they – with – the current - are
4. live - such as - seabirds – on – but – and – go to – pelicans – sea - land

1.2.8   Gaptext

Complete the gap text

Many laymen _____ conquering the sea because there is still so much unknown about _____. However research can prove that _____ have an _____ effect. Algae have a versatile biotechnological use such as _____. Sponges are raised in _____ cultures to do research about their pharmaceutical _____.

Sponges which are unable to move are called _____ organisms.

Marine _____ themselves can be used to _____ waste in the sea.

1.2.9   Pictures of Marine Sealife

Create a sentence
See Figs. 1.3 and 1.4

1.2.10 Important Words in the Field of Blue Biotechnology

Nouns	Verbs	Adjectives
aquatic flora – Wasserflora	to differentiate – unterscheiden	aquatic – Wasser
aquatic toxicology – Wassertoxologie	to commercialise – kommerzialisieren	scarce – selten
cultivation of algae – Kultivierung von Algen	to focus on – abzielen auf	unicellular – einzellig
micro-algae – Mikroalgen	to investigate – erforschen	pharmaceutical – pharmazeutisch
metabolite – Stoffwechselprodukt	to indicate – anzeigen	bubbling – blubbernd
commodities – Wirtschaftsgüter	to synthesise – synthetisieren	marketable – marktfähig
mammals – Säugetiere	to advance – voranschreiten	at random – zufällig
molluscs – Weichtiere	to convert into – umwandeln in	efficient – effizient
invertebrates – wirbellose Tiere	to come across sth. – auf etw. stoßen	anti-inflammatory – entzündungshemmend
vertebrates – Wirbeltiere	to adapt – sich anpassen	ex situ – außerhalb der eigentlichen Umgebung

1.3   Green Biotechnology (Tab. 1.4)

Introduction to Green Biotechnology
Green biotechnology mainly deals with the genetic modification of plants to make them more drought resistant or to strengthen certain characteristic traits to receive a better **yield** or to make them resistant to viral diseases. Furthermore it also stands for the development of **biopesticides** and **biofertilizers** to reduce the chemical impact of nitrogen on the environment.

Breeding hybrids is a further field of green biotechnology e.g. tomatoes are more long-living than normal tomatoes due to hybridization. Green biotechnology is the topic which is discussed about worldwide due to ethical and moral issues.

Tab. 1.4 Vocabulary for the introduction to green biotechnology

English	German
yield	Ausbeute
biopesticides	Biopestizide
biofertilizers	Biodünger
breeding	Züchtung

Tandempartner A
Find the right words for the marine sealife pictures,
partner B has the right answer:
For example:

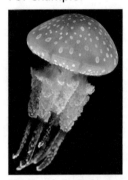

Name: Jelly fish.

Sentence: A jelly fish is luminiscent.

Now it is your turn, Partner A:

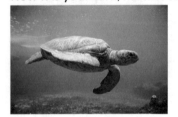

Name: _____

Sentence: _____

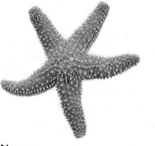

Name: _____
Sentence: _____

Solution for the pictures of Partner B:

Name of the picture 1: algae - Algae have a versatile use in blue biotechnology.

Name of the picture 2: St. James scallop – Sea shells/St. James Scallops can be found on the beach.

Name of the picture 3: a sea gull – A sea gull lives at the shores. (Bild von Capri23auto auf Pixabay)

Fig. 1.3 Tandempartner A

Now it is your turn, Tandempartner B

Find the right words of the marine sea life for the following pictures. Partner A has the right answer.

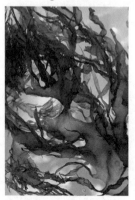

Name: _____

Sentence: _____

Name: _____

Sentence:_____

Name: _____

Sentence:_____

Solution of the name of the pictures from Partner A:

Name of the picture 1: Jelly fish. A jelly fish is luminiscent.

Name of the picture 2: Sea turtle. A sea turtle lives a long time.

Name of the picture 3: Star fish. A star fish is loved by everyone.

Fig. 1.4 Tandempartner B

1.3.1   General Text (Tab. 1.5)

Tab. 1.5 Vocabulary for the text: with an eye on hunger, scientists promise in genetic tinkering of plants

English	German
bold	schwungvoll
to tinker	an etw. tüfteln
outfit	Ausstattung
to alleviate	lindern
genetic engineering technique	Gentechnologie
to eke sth. out	sich etw. erkämpfen
borne out	weiter getragen von
traction	Beförderung
gene-altered crops	genverändertes Getreide
plots	Fläche
billed equation	angekündigte Gleichung
genetic alteration	genetische Veränderung
to incorporate	aufnehmen
thale cress	Ackerschmalwand
mouse ear cress	Hornkraut
strains	Stämme
yield	Ausbeute
assembly line	Fließband
cassava	Maniok
cowpeas	Langbohnen
dietary staples	Hauptnahrungsmittel
gene-altered crops	genetisch verändertes Getdeicde
assume	annehmen
resilient	widerstandsfähig

With an Eye on Hunger, Scientists See Promise in Genetic Tinkering of Plants

URBANA, I11. – A decade ago, agricultural scientists at the University of Illinois suggested a **bold** approach to improve the food supply: **tinker** with photosynthesis, the chemical reaction powering nearly all life on Earth.

The idea was greeted skeptically in scientific circles and ignored by funding agencies. But one **outfit** with deep pockets, the Bill and Melinda Gates Foundation, eventually paid attention, hoping the research might help **alleviate** global poverty.

Now, after several years of work funded by the foundation, the scientists are reporting a remarkable result.

Using **genetic engineering techniques** to alter photosynthesis, they increased the productivity of a test plant – tobacco – by as much as 20 %, they said Thursday in a study published by the journal Science. That is a huge number, given that plant breeders struggle **to eke out** gains of 1 or 2 % more conventional approaches.

The scientists have no interest in increasing the production of tobacco; their plan is to try the same alterations in food crops, and one of the leaders of the work believes production gains of 50 % or more may ultimately be achievable. If the **prediction is borne out** in further research – it could take a decade, if not longer, to know for sure – the result might be nothing less than a transformation of global agriculture.

The findings could also intensify the political struggle over genetic engineering of the food supply. Some groups oppose it, arguing that researchers are playing God by moving genes from one species to another. That argument has gained some **traction** with the public, in part because the benefits of **gene-altered crops** have so far been modest at best.

But gains of 40 or 50 % in food production would be an entirely different matter, potentially offering enormous benefits for the world's poorest people, many of them farmers working small **plots** of land in the developing world.

"We're here because we want to alleviate poverty," said Katherine Kahn, the officer at the Gates Foundation overseeing the grant for the Illinois research. "What is it the farmers need, and how can we help them get there?"

One of the leaders of the research, Stephen P. Long, a crop scientist who holds appointments at the University of Illinois at Urbana-Champaign and at Lancaster University in England, emphasized in an interview that a long road lay ahead before any results from the work might reach farmers' fields.

But Dr. Long is also convinced that genetic engineering could ultimately lead to what he called a "second Green Revolution" that would produce huge gains in food production, like the original Green Revolution of the 1960s and 1970s, which transferred advanced agricultural techniques to some developing countries and led to reductions in world hunger.

The research involvers photosynthesis, in which plants use carbon dioxide from the air and energy from sunlight to form new, energy-rich carbohydrates. These compounds are, in turn, the basic energy supply for almost all animal cells, including those of humans. The mathematical description of photosynthesis is sometimes **billed** as "the **equation** that powers the world."

For a decade, Dr. Long had argued that photosnythesis was not actually very efficient. In the course of evolution, several experts said, Mother Nature had focused on the survival and reproduction of plants, not on putting out the maximum amount of seeds or fruits for humans to come along and pick.

Dr. Long thought crop yields might be improved by certain genetic changes. Other scientists doubted it would work, but with the Science paper, Dr. Lang and his collaborator – Krishan K. Niyogi who holds appointments at the University of California, Berkeley, and the Lawrence Berkeley National Laboratory – have gone a long way toward proving their point.

Much of the work at the University of Illinois was carried out by two young researchers from abroad who hold positions in Dr. Long's laboratory, Johannes Kromdijk of the Netherlands and Katarzyna Glowacka of Poland.

No one plans to eat tobacco, of course, nor does the Gates Foundation have any interest in increasing the production of that health-damaging crop. But the researchers used it because tobacco is a particularly fast and easy plant in which to try new **genetic alterations** to see how well they work.

In a recent interview here, Dr. Kromdijk and Dr. Glowacka showed off tiny tobacco plants **incorporating** the genetic changes and described their aspirations.

"We hope it translates into food crops in the way we've shown in tobacco," Dr. Kromodijk said. "Of course, you only know when you actually try it."

In the initial work, the researchers transferred genes from a common laboratory plant, known as thale cress or mouse-ear cress, into **strains** of tobacco. The effect was not to introduce alien substances, but rather to increase the level of certain proteins that already existed in tobacco.

When plants receive direct sunlight, they are often getting more energy than they can use, and they activate a mechanism that helps them shed it as heat – while slowing carbohydrate production. The genetic changes the researchers introduced help the plant turn that mechanism off faster once the excessive sunlight ends, so that the machinery of photosynthesis can get back more quickly to maximal production of carbohydrates.

It is a bit like a factory worker taking a shorter coffee break before getting back to the **assembly line**. But the effect on the overall growth of the tobacco plants was surprisingly large.

When the scientists grew the newly created plants in fields at the University of Illinois, they achieved **yield** increases of 13.5 % in one strain, 19 % in a second and 20 % in a third, over normal tobacco plants grown for comparison.

Because the machinery of photosynthesis in many of the world's food crops is identical to that of tobacco, theory suggests that a comparable manipulation of those crops should increase production. Work is planned to test that in crops that are especially important as dietary staples in Africa, like **cowpeas**, rice and **cassava.**

Two outside experts not involved in the research both used the word "exciting" to describe it. But they emphasized that the researchers had not yet proved that the food supply could be increased.

"How does it look in rice or corn or wheat or sugar beets?" said L. Val Giddings, a senior fellow at the Information Technology and Innovation Foundation in Washington and a longtime advocate of **gene-altered crops**. "You've got to get into a handful of the important crops before you can show this is real and it's going to have a huge impact. We are not there yet."

Barry D. Bruce of the University of Tennessee at Knoxville, who studies photosynthesis, pointed out that the genetic alteration might behave differently in crops where only parts of the plant, such as seeds or fruits, are harvested. In tobacco, by contrast, the entire aboveground plant is harvested – Dr. Bruce called it "a leafy green plant used for cigars!"

Dr. Bruce also noted that, now that the principle has been established, it might be possible to find plant varieties with the desired traits and introduce the changes into crops by conventional breeding, rather than by genetic engineering. Dr. Long and his group agreed this might be possible.

The genetic engineering approach, if it works, may well be used in commercial seeds produced by Western agricultural companies. One of them, Snygenta, has already signed a deal to get a first look at the results. But the Gates Foundation is determined to see the technology, **assuming** its early promise is **borne out**, make its way to African farmers at low cost.

The work is, in part, an effort to secure the food supply against the possible effects of future climate change. If rising global temperatures cut the production of food, human society could be destabilized, but more efficient crop plants could potentially make the food system more **resilient**, Dr. Long said.

"We're in a year when commodity prices are very low, and people are saying the world doesn't need more food," Dr. Long said. "But if we don't do this now, we may not have it when we really need it."

1.3.2   General Questions

1. Describe at least two advantages and disadvantages of green biotechnology!
2. Would you buy GM tomatoes? Give reasons for or against it!
3. Explain the process of photosynthesis!
4. Elucidate how they changed the process of photosynthesis!
5. Draw a conclusion!

1.3.3   Expressing Your Opinion

Agreement	Disagreement	Objection	Opinion

Complete the table with useful phrases expressing your statement.

e.g. for agreement – I couldn't agree more …

for disagreement – I completely disagree …

for objection – I see your point but your arguments are out of proportion …

for opinion – To my point of view …

Divide the class into four groups, discuss the following topics:

1. transgenic microbes
2. transgenic plants
3. cloning
4. gene therapy

One person moderates the discussion by asking questions. The others are divided into the pro group and the contra group.

Act out the discussion. Make sure that you talk freely.

1.3.4   Create a Word Snake

Find a word that has to do with green biotechnology. Restart with the last letter of the word with a new word that is related to green biotechnology.

E.g. **alteresilient**

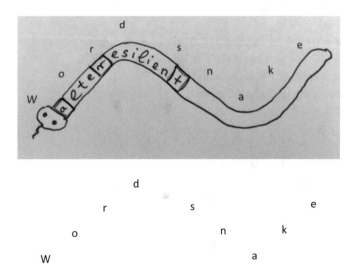

1.3.5   Grammar

Form the questions for the following answers. Ask for the underlined words.

1. I haven't seen him **for ages**.
2. He did his **PhD** in 2009.
3. Photosynthesis was not actually **efficient**.
4. Photosynthesis is often called "**the equation that powers the world**."
5. He gave the article to **Bob**.
6. This article is **the work** of James.
7. We are here because we want **to alleviate poverty**.

8. **These compounds** are the basic energy for all cells.
9. **A long road** lay ahead before any results could be presented.
10. **He opposed** the trial because of his experience.

1.3.6   Translate the Phrases from German into English

1. Ich denke der Autor möchte, dass der Leser …
2. Soweit mir bekannt ist …
3. Ich kann nicht verleugnen …
4. Es gibt mehrere Gründe für …
5. Nach meinem Standpunkt …
6. Wenn wir die Argumente näher betrachten …
7. Um es auf den Punkt zu bringen …
8. Ein gutes Beispiel für …
9. Dieses Beispiel veranschaulicht …
10. Es fällt mir schwer …

1.3.7   Apply Five Sentences Used from Sect. 1.3.6 to the Text

1.3.8   Complete the Sentences

Green technology means to me….

Research in green technology comprises…..

I could – I couldn't imagine to work in the field of green biotechnology because…

Regarding the previous text I come to the conclusion that….

To patent GMO is for me…..

1.3.9   Important Vocabulary for Green Biotechnology

Nouns	Verbs	Adjectives
genetic engineering – Gentechnik	to harness – nutzbar machen	abiotic – abiotisch
biopesticides – Biounkrautvernichtungsmittel	to harvest – ernten	biotic – biotisch
propagation – Vermehrung	to alleviate – lindern	dietary – Nahrungs-
transgenic plants – transgene Pflanzen	to breed – züchten	alien – fremd
genetically – modified organisms (GMO) genetisch veränderte Organismen	to incorporate – einbauen	resilient – widerstandsfähig
alteration – Veränderung	to map – verzeichnen	genetically-modified – genetisch verändert
hybrid – Kreuzung	to alter – verändern	pest-resistant – unkrautresistent
cross-pollination – Fremdbestäubung	to provide – zur Verfügung stellen	beneficial – vorteilshaft
outcrossing – Auskreuzung	to supply – liefern	low-cost – preisgünstig
pest – Unkraut	to tinker – an etw. tüfteln	gene-altered – genverändert

1.4   White Biotechnology

White biotechnology deals with the use of biotechnological processes to produce food or drinks. For bread you need yeast, for wine you need fermentation. White biotechnology is nothing new but one of the ancient techniques of mankind. However the innovative aspect about white biotechnology is the fact that it is made more environmentally friendly. You use in your washing agents or washing powder enzymes that reduce the energy consumption. Since fossil fuels are running out, white biotechnology is becoming more and more important on an industrial scale.

The following text gives you an insight:

1.4.1 General Text (Tab. 1.6)

Tab. 1.6 Vocabulary for the text: white biotechnology

English	German
sustainable	nachhaltig
viability	Lebensfähigkeit
landfills	Deponien
surfactants	Tenside
manifold	vielseitig
sound	gesund
biodegradable	biologisch abbaubar
bacterial strains	Bakterienstämme
to encode sth.	etw. verschlüsseln
et al. – et ali	und andere
reluctant	ungern
viable	lebensfähig
impasse	Sackgasse
resilience	Widerstandsfähigkeit
TM – trademark	Handelsmarke
roadblocks	Hürden
starch	Stärke
herbicides	Unkrautvernichtungsmittel
fertilizers	Düngemittel
irrigation	Bewässerung
feedstock	Rohstoff
stakeholder Interessens	verhretes
regulatory	behördlich
subsidies	Subventionen
advocate	sich für etw. einsetzen
deprived	benachteiligt
impact	Einfluss
to sequester	absondern
committed to	engagiert für
propensity	Neigung
cautious	vorsichtig
adventurous	abenteuerlustig
regulatory	behördlich
paved	geebnet
mature	reif
contender	Herausforderer
feedstock	Rohstoff
stakeholder	Interessensvertreter
subsidies	Subventionen
to advocate sth.	etw. empfehlen

White Biotechnology

The application of biotechnology to industrial production holds many promises for **sustainable** development, but many products still have to pass the test of economic **viability.**

For tens of thousands of years, humans relied on nature to provide them with all the things they needed to make themselves more comfortable. They wove clothes and fabrics from wool, cotton or silk, dyed them with colours derived from plants and animals. Trees provided the material to build houses, furniture and fittings. But this all changed during the first half of the twentieth century, when organic chemistry developed methods to create many of these products from oil. Oil-derived synthetic polymers, coloured with artificial dyes, soon replaced natural fibres in clothes and fabrics. Plastics rapidly replaced wood and metals in many consumer items, buildings and furniture. However, biology might be about to take revenge on these synthetic, petroleum-based consumer goods. Stricter environmental regulations and the growing mass of non-degradable synthetics in **landfills** have made biodegradable products appealing again. Growing concerns about the dependence on imported oil, particularly in the USA, and the awareness that the world's oil supplies are not limitless are additional factors prompting the chemical and biotechnology industries to explore nature's richness in search of methods to replace petroleum-based synthetics.

An entire branch of biotechnology, known as, white biotechnology is devoted to this. It uses living cells – from yeast, molds, bacteria and plants – and enzymes to synthesize products that are easily degradable, require less energy and create less waste during their production. This is not a recent development: in fact, biotechnology has been contributing to industrial processes for some time. For decades, bacterial enzymes have been used widely in food manufacturing and as active ingredients in washing powders to reduce the amount of artificial **surfactants**. Transgenic *Escherichia coli* are used to produce human insulin in large-scale fermentation tanks. And the first rationally designed enzyme, used in detergents to break down fat, was introduced as early as 1988. The benefits of exploiting natural processes and products are **manifold**: they do not rely on fossil resources, are more energy efficient and their substrates and waste are biologically degradable, which all helps to decrease their environmental impact. Using alternative substrates and energy sources, white biotechnology is already bringing many innovations to the chemical, textile, food, packaging and health care industries. It is no surprise then that academics, industry and policy makers are increasingly interested in this new technology, its economy and its contributions to a **sound** environment, which could make it a credible method for sustainable development.

One of the first goals on white biotechnology's agenda has been the production of **biodegradable** plastics. Over the past 20 years, these efforts have concentrated mainly on polyesters of 3-hydroxydacids (PHAs), which are naturally synthesized by a wide range of bacteria as an energy reserve and carbon source. These compounds have properties similar to synthetic thermoplastics and elastomers from propylene to rubber, but are completely and rapidly degraded by bacteria in soil or water. The most abundant PHA is poly(3-hydroxy-butyrate) (PHB), which bacteria synthesize from acetyl-CoA. Growing on glucose, the bacterium *Ralstonia eutropha* can amass up to 85 % of its dry weight in PHB, which makes this microorganism a miniature bioplastic factory.

A major limitation of the commercialization of such bacterial plastics has always been their cost, as they are 5–10 times more expensive to produce than petroleum-based polymers. Much effort has therefore gone into reducing production costs through the development of better **bacterial strains**, but recently a potentially friendly alternative emerged, namely the modification of plants to synthesize PHAs. A small amount of PHB was first produced in *Arabidopsis thaliana* after the introduction of *R. eutropha* genes **encoding two** enzymes that are essential for the conversion of acetyl-CoA to PHB (Poirier **et al.** 1992). Monsanto (St. Louis, MO, USA) then improved this process in 1999. Although this new wave of polymers has enormous potential, the timing of its evolution is uncertain. After initial enthusiasm, Monsanto and AstraZeneca (London, UK) abandoned these projects due to cost concerns. "Producing biopolymers from plants is a promising and fascinating scientific challenge," said Yves Poirier from the Laboratory of Plant Biotechnology at the Institute of Ecology, University of Lausanne, Switzerland. He thinks that companies are **reluctant** to pursue these projects because they need long-term investments that do not meet the companies' financial and time schedules. "Further genetic modifications still need to be introduced in the plants for their improvement," he said, "and once these plants are created, they will require specific harvesting and treatment protocols, with respect to regular plants. All this translates into heavy investments in new infrastructures and processing systems and into a considerable amount of time." Eight to ten years is his rough estimate of how long it will be before plant-produced PHAs might become economically **viable.**

Plans to manufacture a T-shirt from corn sugar have reached the same **impasse.** Dupont (Wilmington, DE, USA), the company that invented nylon, has for many years been developing a polymer based on 1,3-propanediol (PDO), with new levels of performance, **resilience** and softness. Adding an environmentally responsible dimension to the production, Dupont's polymerization plant in Decatur, Illinois (USA) has now successfully manufactured PDO from corn sugar, a renewable resource.

But although their corn-based polymer, called Sorona R, is more environmentally friendly and has improved characteristics, it is again up to the markets to make it a success. "The company plans an effective shift from the petroleum-based production to the bio-based one," said Ian Hudson, Sorona R Business Director at Dupont, "but this will happen if the economic process and market demands justify the transition."

Cargil Dow (Minnetonka, MN, USA) has gone a step further. The company has developed an innovative biopolymer, NatureWorks **TM**, which can be used to manufacture items such as clothing, packaging and office furnishings. The polymer is derived from lactic acid, which is obtained from the fermentation of corn sugar. It has already been brought to the market effectively and has recently appeared in US grocery stores as a container for organic food.

Another product that could benefit greatly from innovative biotechnology is paper. Much of the cost and considerable pollution involved in the paper-making process is caused by 'krafting', a method for removing lignin from the wood substrate. Lignin is the second most abundant polymer in nature after cellulose and provides structural stability to plants. In view of the significant economic benefits that might be achieved, many research efforts went into reducing the amount of lignin or modifying lignin structure in trees, while preserving their growth and structural integrity. Genetically modified trees with these properties already exist (Hu et al. 1999; Chabannes et al. 2001; Li et al. 2003), but money will probably not be made from them anytime soon. Although the paper industry could make a considerable profit by reducing production costs, no large projects in this direction have yet been undertaken. Alain Boudet, Professor at the Centre for Vegetable Biotechnology at the University Paul Sabatier (Castanet-Tolosan, France), identified two major **roadblocks** for the commercialization of transgenic wood. "First of all, trees with altered lingin will need more tests on their actual field performance outside the laboratory before being widely used," he explained. "Secondly, and with much more difficulty, it will be necessary to conquer the public's acceptance to yet new transgenic organisms and to the distribution of products deriving from them."

White biotechnology also concentrates on the production of energy from renewable resources and biomasses. **Starch** from corn, potatoes, sugar cane and wheat is already used to produce ethanol as substitute for gasoline – Henry Ford's first car ran on ethanol. Today, some motor fuel sold in Brazil is pure ethanol derived from sugar cane, and the rest has 20 % ethanol content. In the USA, 10 % of all motor fuel sold is a mixture of 90 % petrol and 10 % ethanol. According to the Organisation for Economic Co-operation and Development's 2001 report on biotechnology and industrial sustainability, the USA now has 58 fuel plants, which produce almost 6 billion litres of ethanol per year.

But turning starch into ethanol is neither the most environmentally nor economically efficient method, as growing plants for ethanol production involves the use of **herbicides**, pesticides, **fertilizers, irrigation** and machinery. Companies such as Novzymes (Bagsward, Denmark), Genencor (Palo Alto, CA, USA) and Madygen (Redwood City, CA, USA) are therefore exploring avenues to derive ethanol specifically from celluloid material in wood, grasses and, more attractively, agricultural waste. Much of their effort is concentrated on developing more effective bacterial cellulases that can break down agricultural waste into simple sugars to create a more plentiful and cheaper raw substrate for the production of ethanol.

Hopeful visionaries have already started to talk about a 'carbohydrate economy' replacing the old 'hydrocarbon economy'. However, "making biomass an effective **feedstock** is not a cheap process," reminded Kirsten Staer, Director of **Stakeholder** Communications at Novozymes. To get the production of biofuel up and running on a commercial basis, alongside the development of new feedstock collection systems and the creation of special production plants, a different pricing of biofuel will be required, she commented. "The price structure for fossil fuel is fixed in the market by **regulatory** frameworks. If the biofuel production is to be successful, it will be necessary to enforce policies that introduce **subsidies** to bioethanol production, for instance, or put taxes on fossil fuel production," Staer said.

This has not stopped J. Craig Venter from founding the Institute for Biological Energy Alternatives (IBEA) in Rockville, Maryland (USA) last year to **advocate** the production of cleaner forms of energy. IBEA recently received a US 53 million grant from the US Department of Energy, primarily to engineer an artificial microorganism to produce hydrogen. **Deprived** of the genes for sugar formation that normally use hydrogen ions, this organism could devote all of its energies to the production of excess hydrogen and, ideally, become a synthetic energy producer.

White biotechnology may also benefit medicine and agriculture. Vitamin B 2 (riboflavin), for instance, is widely used in animal feed, human food and cosmetics and has traditionally been manufactured in a six-step chemical process. At BASF (Ludwigshafen, Germany) more than 1000 tonnes of vitamin B2 are now produced per year in a single fermentation. Using the fungus Ahsbya gossypii as a biocatalyst, BASF achieved an overall reduction in cost and environmental **impact** of 40 %. Similarly, cephalexin, an antibiotic that is active against Gram-negative bacteria and is normally produced in a lengthy ten-step chemical synthesis, is now produced in a shorter fermentation-based process at DSM Life Sciences Products (Heerlen, The Netherlands). However, vitamin B2 is just a single success story – other vitamins and drugs are still cheaper to produce with classic organic chemistry than by innovative white biotechnology.

Nevertheless, the potential environmental benefits of shifting to biofeedstocks and bioprocesses are substantial, thinks Wolfgang Jenseit from the Institute for Applied Ecology (Freiburg, Germany). "The new bioproduction processes substitute complex chemistry reactions. This, of course, corresponds to significant energy and water savings" he explained. It also benefits the atmosphere: the carbon needed to make bioethanol from biomass was **sequestered** by plants from the atmosphere, so putting it back by burning ethanol does not add to global warming. Jenseit pointed out. This is certainly good news for the countries that **committed to** limiting greenhouse-gas emissions by ratifying the Kyoto treaty.

And the economic benefits are expected to follow. According to the global consultancy firm McKinsey & Company, white biotechnology will occupy up to 10–20 % of the entire chemical market in 2010, with annual growth rates of Euro 11–22 billion. Huge differences exist, however, in the ways white biotechnology is managed in Europe and the USA, says Jens Riese, a Frankfurt-based Principal Associate at McKinsey & Company. "First of all, the overall sum invested in the US in the white biotech business is 250 million USDollar, a sum which by far exceeds the total European investment", he said. "Probably driven by a stronger geopolitical will of becoming independent from fossil fuel import, the US has shown a clearer **propensity** in the development of such technologies. Europe, on the other hand, is culturally more **cautious** and less **adventurous** in accepting innovative methodologies."

But white biotechnology has drawn interest in Europe. "There is consciousness about the need for innovation in this direction," said Oliver Wolf, Scientific Officer at the Institute for Prospective Technological Studies in Seville, Spain. "Although as yet no specific legislation exists, important steps are being taken towards the promotion of white biotechnology in Europe." White biotechnology has potentially large benefits, both economically and environmentally for a wide range of applications. The way for its development is being paved, but it remains a relatively young technology that has to compete with a **mature** oil-based chemical industry that has had nearly a century to optimize its methods and production processes. Nevertheless, the growing concerns about the environment and the possibility of cheaper oil in the future make white biotechnology a serious **contender.**

1.4.2   General Questions

1. Find a headline for each paragraph of the text.
2. State at least three innovations of white biotechnology, describe them more closely.
3. Clarify what problems go along with new white biotechnological inventions?
4. Exemplify the reasons for the environmentally-friendliness of white biotechnology.
5. Some adversaries say that biofuel is not environmentally-friendly. Give reasons for this statement.
6. Illustrate the success of white biotechnology. Find arguments for your statement.
7. Comment on the differences between the USA and Europe regarding white biotechnology.

1.4.3 Grammar

Decide whether the following "-ing"-forms are participles or gerunds, give reasons and translate the sentence into German.

1. **Growing** concern on the dependence on imported oil makes white biotechnology attractive.
2. The awareness that oil supplies are not limitless are factors **prompting** the biotechnology industry to explore nature's richness.
3. Biotechnology **has been contributing** to industrial processes for some time.
4. Bacterial enzymes have widely been used for the food **manufacturing**.
5. The benefits of **exploiting** natural processes are manifold.
6. Much effort has therefore gone into **reducing** production costs.
7. **Producing** biopolymers from plants is a scientific challenge.
8. The company **having** invented nylon **has** for many years **been developing** a polymer with new levels of performance, resilience and softness.
9. Many research efforts went into **reducing** the amount of lignin.
10. Trees with altered lignin will need more tests outside the laboratory before **being** widely used.

1.4.4 Find the Words

Ten words from the text are hidden. Can you find them all?

```
S M X Z A P U R T C O M M I T T E D F
C R E L U C T A N T U A L M C R A V L
O O S Z Y I L A N D F I L L U M A C I
N A X T O S F R M L U M R S T U L K M
T D F X U O U V M B E P A E F R S U A
E B C A I U I K Y M T A R U V A C B N
N L X N U N R V K R X C V L M N X Z I
D O C B S D T K L S R T X S N F R D F
E C X M S R X M A T U R E X T U V U O
R K A P S T A K E H O L D E R I M E L
S X U T N A U Z Y S M V U T A R S C D
E N C O D E B I O D E G R A D A B L E
```

1.4.5   Complete the Prefix Bio- with Ten Complete Words

E.g. bio-fuel

bio	bio
bio	bio
bio	bio
bio	bio
bio	bio

1.4.6   Match the Word

Can you categorize the words from Sect. 1.4.5 into a field of the colours of biotechnology? Match the word to the ten categories of biotechnology.

E.g. biofuel belongs to the category of green biotechnology.
E.g. bioluminescent belongs to no category
E.g. bioactive belongs to all categories

1.4.7   Complete the Table

	Red biotechnology	Blue biotechnology	Green biotechnology	White biotechnology
Main concern				
Main differences				
Main advantages				
I could imagine working in the field of..... because...				

1.4.8   Quiz About the Colours of Biotechnology

Repetition of the vocabulary of red, blue, green and white biotechnology:
Red biotechnology – Blue biotechnology – Green biotechnology – White biotechnology

100	100	100	100
80	80	80	80
60	60	60	60
40	40	40	40
20	20	20	20

Divide the class into two groups. The teacher names five German words in the four fields. The pupils have to translate them into English.

The most difficult word has 100 points. The less difficult one has 20 points.

The winner is who has most words right.

1.4.9   Important Words in the Field of White Biotechnology

Noun	Verb	Adjective
biodegradability – biologische Abbaubarkeit	to apply – anwenden	biodegradable – biologisch abbaubar
biofuel – Biobrennstoff	to prompt – veranlassen	environmentally-friendly – umweltfreundlich
biopowerplant – Biogaskraftwerk	to devote – verwenden	appealing – ansprechend
biopurification system – Bioreinigungssystem	to synthesize – synthetisieren	bacterial – bakteriell
catalysts – Katalysatoren	to contribute – dazu beitragen	rationally – rational
destruction of hazardous chemicals – Zerstörung gefährlicher Chemikalien	to catalyse – katalysieren	energy-efficient – energieeffizient
pollutant disposal – Schadstoffbeseitigung	to concentrate – sich darauf konzentrieren	increasingly – ansteigend
polluters-pays-principle – Verursacherprinzip	to degrade – abbauen	abundant – im Überfluss
sewage treatment – Abwasserbehandlung	to amass up sth. – etw. anhäufen	bioplastic – bioplastisch
waste compost plant – Abfallkompostanlage	remediate – beseitigen, sanieren	scientific – wissenschaftlich

1.5   Grey Biotechnology (Tab. 1.7)

Introduction to Grey Biotechnology
Grey biotechnology comprises all biotechnological procedures which are used for the preparation of drinking water, the purification of **sewage**, the restoration of **contaminated** grounds or the cleaning of **exhaust gases**. The procedure applied is mostly the fermentation that is the enzymatic transformation of organic substances. In other words grey biotechnology is concerned with the removal of pollutants and environmental biotechnology.

1.5.1   General Text

Grey Biotechnology – A Chance for Efficient Waste Management
Grey biotechnology is an environmentally friendly way to remove contaminants by using microorganisms such as fungi, protozoa, bacteria, algae and viruses from water or soil.

Around 140 million tonnes of synthetic polymers are produced each year. It takes centuries to decay them. The water pollution in seas and oceans is immense.

Therefore grey biotechnology is a real chance to treat contaminated soil, oil spillage and radioactive contamination.

Scientists have developed bacteria eating plastics (named Ideonella sakaiensis 201-F6).

Grey biotechnology is also used to protect indigenous fauna which is threatened by foreign plants called phytoremediation.

It is also used to remake former brownfields by enhancing bacterial degradation of contaminants and adding nutrients to the soil. This procedure is called bioremediation.

However it is not applicable for soil that contains cadmium or lead.

A simple application of grey biotechnology is your compost in the garden.

Tab. 1.7 Vocabulary for the introduction to grey biotechnology

English	German
sewage	Abwasser
contaminated	verunreinigt
exhaust gases	Abgase

1.5.2   General Questions

1. Give at least three applications of bioremediation.
2. Explain the advantage and disadvantage of bioremediation.
3. Find differences between white and grey biotechnology.

1.5.3   Shortened Relative Clauses

Match the sentences together by using an "–ing"- form:

1. Bioremediation is also applied to contaminated wastewater. It cleans the contaminated wastewater without aggressive chemicals.
2. Nutrients are added to the soil. It enhances degradation of contaminants.
3. Bioremediation is not a feasible strategy at sites with high concentrations of chemicals. These chemicals contain lead.
4. Bioremediation take advantage of the metabolic process. It can degrade concentration of different contaminants.
5. The process of bioremediation involves the introduction of new organisms. It enhances the degradation rate of indigenous fauna.

1.5.4   Explain the Following Words:*

1. protozoa
2. effluents
3. oil spills
4. feasible
5. phytoremediation

1.5.5   Draw an Advertisement for Bioremediation

Imagine you work for a company which main focus is bioremediation.
Draft an advertisement for their webpage.

1.5.6   What Is the Up-to-date Value of Bioremediation According to You?

How often is bioremediation applied? What is your estimation?

1.5.7 Complete the Gap Text

1. _____ biotechnological purification chemical cleaning was used.
2. Water which is not clean is called _____.
3. Toxic materials are also called _____.
4. Not every biotechnological theory can be _____ in practice.
5. Legal authorities can _____ the use of bioremediation.

1.5.8 Think About More Uses of Bioremediation than the Text States!

1.5.9 Important Vocabulary in the Field of Grey Biotechnology

Noun	Verb	Adjective
purification – Reinigung	to remediate – beseitigen	enzymatic – enzymatisch
sewage – Abwasser	bioremediate – biosanieren	feasible – machbar
restoration – Sanierung	to hasten – sich beeilen	indigenous – einheimisch
contamination – Verunreinigung	to recover sth. – etw. zurückgewinnen	aerobic – aerob
exhaust gases – Abgase	to discharge – entlassen	anaerobic – anaerob
adjustment – Angleichung	to apply to – anwenden	metabolic – metabolisch
pollutants – Verunreiniger	to pose – etw. darstellen	accidental – zufällig
bioremediation – Biosanierung	to take advantage of – einen Vorteil haben/etw. ausnutzen	uncommon – ungewöhnlich
degradation rate – Abbaurate	to recycle – wieder verwerten	regulatory – behördlich
effluents – Abwässer	to perform – etw. durchführen	toxic – giftig

1.6 Yellow Biotechnology

Yellow biotechnology develops products for application in green, red and white biotechnology. E.g. it fights off pests on an environmentally friendly way by using peptides (green biotechnology) or it develops the inhibition of resistant antibiotics (red biotechnology). Furthermore it harnesses enzymes for the production of glutenfree food (white biotechnology). The name yellow derives from the substance hemolymph which is a substance similar to blood in insects and is yellow. Basically yellow biotechnology is concerned with food production.

Tab. 1.8 Vocabulary for the text: yellow biotechnology application on the food industry through in vitro cell culture meats

English	German
pervasive	allgegenwärtig
foodies	Feinschmecker
daunting	abschreckend
bovine	Rinder
to remedy sth.	abhelfen
toll	Gebühr

1.6.1 General Text (Tab. 1.8)

Yellow Biotechnology Application on the Food Industry Through In Vitro Cell Culture Meats

As mentioned in our previous article, the biotechnology industry can be broken down into color categories based on the techniques or products involved in that sector. For example, blue biotechnology includes practices utilizing ocean resources, whereas red biotechnology is related to pharmaceutical products or biomedical engineering. Yellow biotechnology involves the use of bio-engineering to make food. A classic example of yellow biotech's adaption of natural resources for our palates is brewing beer – harnessing the natural yeast fermentation process to fuel college fraternities and connoisseurs alike.

A current hot topic within the food industry and culture and therefore yellow biotech, is sustainability. It is well known that the meat industry, in particular, has a drastic, and **pervasive**, effect on local and global environments.[1] This damaging effect results from resource diversion used to create farms, as well as the subsequent byproducts and run off from their existence.[2]

Deforestation, clean water usage, and heavy feed requirements are necessary to raise the livestock, while antibiotics, pesticides, animal waste, and hormones directly pollute land and water to maintain them. The meat industry overall is responsible, for up to 24 % of greenhouse gas emissions, with no sign of slowing down.[3] Despite the implications for both human health and the environment, meat demand is increasing even as our natural resources are diminishing.

However, from great demand comes great potential. Within the yellow biotech sector, biologists and **foodies** are rising to the challenge. One exciting company, founded by Dr. Mark Post, uses *in vitro* cell culture techniques on adult cow stem cells to manufacture **bovine** muscle tissue – aka hamburger meat. The end result lowers land use by up to 99 %, water use by 96 %, and greenhouse gas emissions by 96 % when compared to other animal meat products.[4] Dr. Post conducted this research at Maastricht University, Netherlands, and live aired the first tasting of his "test tube meat" made up of over 20,000 hand-cultured muscle strands. In August 2013, taste testers noted the lack of fat or juiciness, but gave full points for the mouth feel and definitively preferred the *in vitro* meat to a vegetable-based substitute.

Since then, Dr. Post has taken his technology towards the market with his company MosaMeat. The cost of the first hamburger was a **daunting** Euro 250,000 (over USD 311,000). According to the company however, many of these costs were due to standard academic laboratory fees and the overall cost of operating at such a small scale. Ideally, this could be **remedied** by scaling up production and further refining their growth process. Considering the company plans to go global to help fill the hunger gap, achieving efficiencies of scale is very much a part of their long term plans. Still, the company has a few things to work out moving forward on the science end. The current culture system requires fetal bovine serum to grow the cells into functional supplement used daily in cell culture labs, for a company intent on using as minimal animal products with the smallest environmental impact possible, the question remains if a synthetic serum might be able to take its place.

Overall, MosaMeat and other *in vitro* meat companies show huge potential and have momentum on their side. With the current rate of research and initial progress shown, both environmentalists and animal lovers, as cheap, sustainable hamburger on the table, without the costs to the animals or environment.

To see where *in vitro* meat might take us in the future, check out this website for Bistro in vitro. While none of the menu is available as of today, they show there's no limit to the possibilities that this new technology could bring – and that it may be closer to your menu you think.

1. Herrero M et al (2013) Biomass use, production, feed efficiencies, and greenhouse gas emissions from global livestock systems. Proc Natl Acad Sci 110:20888–20893
2. Scheer R, Moss D (2011) How does meat in the diet take an environmental toll? Sci Am 1. https://www.scientificamerican.com/article/me-and-environment/
3. Fiela N (2008) Meeting the demand: an estimation of potential future greenhouse gas emissions from meat production. Ecol Econ 67:412–419
4. Tuomisto HL, Ellis MJ, Haastrup P (2014) Environmental impacts of cultured meat: alternative production scenarios. Environ Sci Technol 14044:6117–6123

1.6.2 General Questions

1. Explain the relationship between sustainability and yellow biotechnology!
2. Would you buy in vitro meat?
3. Evaluate the advantages and disadvantages of in vitro meat.
4. Do you think it is realistic in the future?
5. Find a headline for each paragraph!

1.6.3 Vocabulary for Commenting Texts

Translate the German sentences into English.

1. Ich muss dem Autor widersprechen …
2. Es ist fraglich …
3. Das ändert jedoch nichts daran …
4. Man könnte entgegnen, dass …
5. Wenn man das Für und Wider abwägt, komme ich zu der Schlussfolgerung …
6. Soweit ich es beurteilen kann…
7. Ich bin geteilter Meinung …
8. Lassen Sie mich ein Beispiel anführen …
9. Mein Eindruck von dem Text ist …
10. Zusammenfassend lässt sich sagen …

Use at least five phrases from 1 to 10 for drawing a conclusion about the text.

1.6.4 Linking Words

To comment texts linking words emphasize your versatility:
First translate the linking words:

1 trotz	11 offensichtlich
2 obwohl	12 während
3 eigentlich	13 als Tatsache
4 darüber hinaus	14 außerdem
5 als Erstes	15 um dies weiter zu verfolgen
6 schließlich	16 daher
7 kurz gesagt	17 ebenso wie
8 in Bezug auf	18 zudem
9 im Vergleich	19 zweifellos
10 zusammenfassend	20 im Gegensatz

1.6.5   Linking Words in Use

Use the following topics and make up a sentence with a linking word:

1. Red biotechnology – Alzheimer
   E.g. the analysis of the genetic make up of a person is thus useful for the treatment of Alzheimer.
2. Green biotechnology – crops
3. Blue biotechnology – research of jellyfish
4. White biotechnology – fermentation
5. Grey biotechnology – purification

1.6.6   Tandem

See Figs. 1.5 and 1.6

PARTNER A

You should find the words in the gap texts which are used in the text.

Partner B has the solution.

1. _____ means that the environment is not damaged by using e.g. renewable energy.

2. The damages of men caused environmental destruction is _____

3. _____ are people who love fancy food.

4. You can buy cow milk or _____ milk.

5. This price is really _____.

6. Brewing beer is an example of the use of _____.

7. You can _____ the sun to produce solar energy.

8. I can taste the saltiness on my _____.

9. In future we could _____ real meat by in vitro meat.

10. Greenhouse gas emissions are increasing also because of the _____ of rain forests.

Solution for Partner B:

1. byproduct
2. are running off
3. implications
4. conducted
5. starvation
6. environmentalists
7. the intent
8. in vitro
9. test tube
10. fetal bovine serum

Fig. 1.5 Tandem partner A

PARTNER B

You should find the words in the gap texts which are used in the text.

Partner A has the solution

1. Cream is a _____ of milk.

2. Fossil fuels _____ by the year 2050.

3. Despite the negative _____ of meat production, the meat production is increasing.

4. Maastricht University _____ the research.

5. The long term plan is to stop _____ .

6. _____ are people who are active in the protection of their sourrounding.

7. _____ of the company is to minimize a negative impact on the environment.

8. _____ meat is a good alternative for people who love animals.

9. This artificial meat is also called _____ meat because it is produced in the laboratory.

10. A negative aspect is that you need _____ to produce artificial meat.

Solution for Partner A:

1. sustainability
2. pervasive
3. foodies
4. bovine
5. daunting
6. bioengineering
7. harness
8. palate
9. substitute
10. deforestation

Fig. 1.6 Tandem partner B

1.6.7   Syntax

He gave me a book.
  me = indirect object
  book = direct object
  He called me a fool.
Me = direct object
  Fool = object complement
He was always a good student.
  Good student = subject complement
Decide whether the bold words are a direct object, an indirect object, an object complement or a subject complement.

1. Meat industry has a drastic effect **on local and global environment**.
2. He called this in vitro meat **challenging**.
3. MosaMeat shows huge **potential**.
4. Foodies will be made **curious**.
5. They will give **him more orders**.

1.6.8   Proverbs with Colours

Translate the proverbs.

1. To be between the devil and the deep blue sea.
2. All that glitters is not gold.
3. She is green with envy.
4. That is still a grey area.
5. She was caught red-handed.
6. I tickled pink.
7. I told her a white lie because I didn't want to hurt her.
8. She is yellow-bellied.
9. He blackmailed him.
10. I am always browned off when I see him.
11. He goes gathering orange blossoms.

Find other proverbs with colours by finding corresponding German proverbs in English.

1.6.9   Important Words in the Field of Yellow Biotechnology

Noun	Verb	Adjective
inhibition – Hemmung	to harness – ernten	resistant to – widerstandsfähig gegenüber
yeast fermentation – Hefefermentation	to feed – füttern	pervasive – allgegenwärtig
livestock – Viehbestand	to manufacture – herstellen	in vitro – in vitro
demand – Nachfrage	to lower – vermindern	bovine – Rinder-
foodies – Feinschmecker	to emit – ausstoßen	environmental – Umwelt-
substitute – Ersatz	to substitute – ersetzen	sustainable – nachhaltig
small scale – kleine Skala	to work out – ausarbeiten	current – aktuell
bioengineering – Biotechnik	to involve – einbeziehen	subsequent – nachfolgend
sustainability – Nachhaltigkeit	to fuel – anheizen	vegetable-based – gemüsebasierend
byproduct – Nebenprodukt	to run off – ausgehen	synthetic – synthetisch

1.7   Brown Biotechnology

Brown biotechnology is a very up to date topic as droughts are increasing due to climate change. On the basis of genetically modified plants brown biotechnology deals with the research of drought resistant plants.

1.7.1   General Text (Tab. 1.9)

Tab. 1.9 Vocabulary for the text: GMO crops could help stem famine and future global conflicts

English	German
floods	Überschwemmungen
drought	Dürre
myriad	unzählig
to trigger	auslösen
to withstand	Stand halten
induced	hervorgerufen durch
Impact	Einfluss
teff	Zwerghirse
indigenous	einheimisch
to bounce back	sich wieder erholen von
depriviation	Mangel
non-edible	nicht essbar
dormancy	Winterruhe
to pinpoint	darauf hinweisen
agave plant	Agavenpflanze
to mitigate	lindern

GMO Crops Could Help Stem Famine and Future Global Conflicts

When most of us think about the threats posed by climate change, events like **floods**, **droughts**, intense storms and hotter temperatures come to mind. These are all, according to the vast majority of scientists, exactly what we can expect to see more and more of. However, what is often overlooked are the sociopolitical consequences of these climatic changes, in other words, we tend to view these natural disasters in a vacuum without recognizing the **myriad** ways in which climate change is both directly and indirectly shaping economies, cultures and governments.

This being the case, looking back at conflicts such as those in Syria and the Sudan, it has become increasingly clear that climate change played a role in **triggering** the instability that led to these conflicts. Which begs the question could these conflicts have been prevented through non-political measures that responded to changes in climate?

The answer increasingly seems to be yes. Further developments in biotechnology and a deeper understanding of what triggered the conflicts in Syria and Sudan point to novel prevention solutions grounded in modern agriculture. The arrival of genetically engineered (GE) drought-tolerant crops can **withstand** longer and more intense droughts could have the potential to prevent future conflicts.

Both the conflicts in Syria and the Sudan followed intense, climate change-**induced** drought periods that caused mass crop failures and famine. Beginning as early as 1998 and continuing into the 21st century, Syria and the surrounding region experienced a drought that, according to research published in the Journal of Geophysical Research, was the worst the region had experienced in 900 years.

The subsequent crop failure and famine eventually forced rural populations into urban centers to seek out food and better living conditions. The unfortunate result of this mass migration of people was the failure of Syrian cities to provide basic goods and services, leading to public unrest and eventually conditions ripe for civil war.

Had these farmers been better prepared to deal with years-long drought conditions, might Syria have avoided their civil war? The answer is not clear, as the conflict in Syria is complex and it is impossible to say whether it could have been prevented by any one action.

However, learning from Syria, we can assume that in the future, reducing the **impacts** of drought on particularly at risk populations through implementation of modern farming practices and the introduction of GE drought-tolerant crops could play a major role in preventing political instability.

Though there are few GE drought-tolerant crops on the market today, scientists all over the world are developing new crops in an effort to better prepare farmers for the increasingly severe droughts we expect to see.

Researchers at the University of Cape Town in South Africa are working to genetically engineer **teff**, an African grain important to many **indigenous** groups, in order to increase its ability **to bounce back** from water **deprivation**. The group intends to pull genes from a **non-edible** native plant, *Myroflammus flabellifolius*, which has the ability to enter **dormancy** during intense drought, but then **bounce back** in the event of rain. Small scale, public projects such as these that **pinpoint** specific crops in specific areas will be the key to combatting the effects of climate change.

Similarly, Xiaophang Yang at the Oakridge National Laboratory in Tennessee is attempting something more ambitious and wide reaching in this research on understanding how naturally drought-resistant plants use a different type of photosynthesis to endure the stressful conditions of drought. Yang's goal is to map the genetics behind **agave plants** method of photosynthesis, which differs from most plants, with the hope of one day introducing those genes into common crops. Not only would this allow for crops to withstand drought conditions, it would also open up new areas for farming that were once too dry.

As the genetic engineering of crops rapidly expands in the public sector, using GMOs as a tool for **mitigating** the effects of climate change will become a more and more potent option, offering hope for feeding a growing global population and serving as a stabilizing force in drought ridden parts of the world.

Josh Winkler is a freelance journalist who focuses on genetic engineering, the **Anthropocerne** *and the outdoors industry.*

1.7.2   General Questions

1. Do you think that droughts and floods can be a cause for war? Give reasons for your statement!
2. Go into detail about the consequences of droughts.
3. Make up your mind about fighting against droughts.
4. Do you think that GMO plants could contribute to fight against hunger? Give reasons for your statement!

1.7.3   Presentation

Present in a group of four a country which is concerned with droughts (Sambia, Mosambique, Botswana, South Africa, India, Chile, South Asia).

1.7.4 Quiz About Droughts

1. What is a continental climate?
   A Course of temperature based on seasons
   B Climate in Europe
   C Climate on land
2. What is meant by hydrological drought?
   A Trees get brown leaves.
   B Water gauge under the normal value.
   C Too few precipitations during one year.
3. What does the El-Niño phenomenon mean?
   A The El-Niño phenomenon leads to floods in South America and droughts in Africa.
   B The wind stream between America and Europe.
   C The rise of water temperature in the oceans.
4. Mega-drought is
   A a drought in a period of one year
   B a drought within a decade
   C a drought within twenty years
5. Dust bowl is a word for
   A a drought period in North America between 1930–38
   B a windstream in Africa
   C a tornado
6. What are isohydric plants?
   A The water contents of tissue is kept up if water deficiency occurs.
   B Plants that can store more water during droughts.
   C Plants which are genetically modified.
7. Turgor is a botanical expression for
   A process which describes the liquid flow of a plant.
   B value to measure the pressure in plants.
   C pressure on the cell wall of a plant containing liquid.
8. Transgenic plants are defined as
   A Plants that are breeded
   B Plants that contain genes which are not originally from them
   C Plants that have completely different colours than the natural ones
9. C4 plants
   A are mostly flowers.
   B cannot survive in hot climate.
   C bind CO_2 better than normal plants.
10. EFSA stands for the abbreviation
   A European Foundation for secure application of GM food
   B European Foundation of standard approvals for GM food
   C European Food Safety Authority

1.7.5   Active and Passive Sentences

Transfer the sentences either into the active or passive form.

1. Researchers at the University of Cape Town are working to genetically engineer teff.
2. What is often overlooked are the sociopolitical consequences of climatic change.
3. Yang's goal is to map the genetics of agave plants.
4. The crop failure forced rural populations into urban centers.
5. The genetic engineering of crops is rapidly being expanded by the public sector.
6. Genetically modified organisms withstand drought conditions.
7. Natural disasters are shaping economies.
8. Scientists all over the world are developing new crops.
9. He followed the rules of the modification of plants.
10. Small scale projects will be the key for combatting droughts.

1.7.6   Find Words in the Text Which Have the Following Meaning

1. The fact that there is not enough to eat.
2. There is some food such as fly agaric which is poisonous and not possible to eat.
3. In Africa people who are natives and born in Africa are called a native group.
4. Due to droughts or floods there is no possibility to harness the crop.
5. Genetically modified crop is able to resist to droughts.

1.7.7   Make Up a Mind Map About Droughts

DROUGHT

1.7.8   Find the Synonyms and Antonyms of the Following Words

synonyms	antonyms
threat	rural
myriad	major
to withstand	severe
to induce	common
indigenous	to expand

1.7.9   Important Words in the Field of Brown Biotechnology

Noun	Verb	Adjective
creation of enhanced seeds – Schaffung von verbessertem Saatgut	to trigger – auslösen	arable – bebaubar
drought – Dürre	to withstand – Stand halten	myriad – vielfältig
flood – Überschwemmung	to engineer – entwickeln	climate-induced – klimabedingt
crop failure – Ernteausfall	to bounce back – wieder auf die Beine kommen	subsequent – hinternanderfolgend
impact – Einfluss	to combat – bekämpfen	ripe – reif
water deprivation – Wassermangel	to endure – anhalten	drought-tolerant – dürretolerant
mitigation – Linderung	to map – verzeichnen	indigenous – einheimisch
yield – Ausbeute	to open up – eröffnen	non-edible – nicht essbar
feeding – Nahrung	to wither – verdörren	stressful – anstrengend
precipitation – Niederschlag	to shrivel – vertrocknen	drought ridden – von Dürre beherrscht

1.8   Violet Biotechnology

Ethics derives from Greek 'ethos' which means custom, habit, character or disposition. Ethics is a set of moral principles, which defines what is good for individuals and society. These principles are influenced by our culture and religion e.g. you must not steal. It comprises aspects such as how to live a good life, what are our rights and responsibilities and the language of right and wrong as well as moral decisions what is good or bad. There are different categories of ethics: metha-ethic concerns the origin of ethical principles. Normative ethics establishes a set of criteria what is right or wrong. Applied ethics is concerned with up to date topics such as children soldiers.

Violet biotechnology takes into consideration ethical and moral issues which occur by the modification of genes and thus leads to the problematic issues such as patent rights.

Tab. 1.10 Vocabulary for the text: thinking ethically about human biotechnology

English	German
sparking	sprühend
to elicit	hervorrufen
to permeate	durchdringen
contentious	umstritten
to constrain	belegen
propensity	Neigung
fatedness	Schicksal
quietistic	quietistisch
captivating	fesselnd
daunting	erschrechend
ramification	Verzweigung
realm	Königreich
incentives	Prämienlohn, Leistungsanreiz
scurried away	weggehuscht
unanticipated	unerwartet
to impede	verhindern
incumbent	obligatorisch
peer-reviewed	durch Fachleute überprüft
savvy	klug, schlau
stakeholder	Interessensvertreter
to inculcate	einprägen
inextricably	untrennbar
inclination	Neigung
to inculcate	einprägen
to err	sich irren
coming to grips with sth.	mit etw. zurecht kommen
trajectories	Abläufe

1.8.1   General Text (Tab. 1.10)

Thinking Ethically About Human Biotechnology

Modern biotechnology, with its focus on molecular biology and its concern for increasing human health and life spans, is all about the future. This biotech future presses in daily, **sparking** imaginations. At the same time, it **elicits** wariness or even fear that humanity is gaining too much power or too little choice over human evolution and destiny. The political climate, **permeated** as it is by a ferocious "moral approach" to science policy, heightens this public concern. We seem to have lost our capacity for rational discourse in the public arena. The biotech industry has increasingly realized that not only regulatory schemes but also **contentious** public and political debate can either enable or **constrain** research and development. For better or worse, science is political.

   We Can, but Must We?

   Since the birth of Dolly the cloned sheep, public concern about advancing biotechnology has been enflamed by the suspicion that science is at the mercy of the technological imperative, the **propensity** to think that because something can be done, it is inevitable. This seemingly easy slide from can to will – because it is technically possible to clone a child into existence, it will become an everyday occurrence, for example – leaves some with a sense of **fatedness**, a sense that science is unstoppable. Hence, for those people, science is not a subject of ethical concern. In this view, at best, ethics takes a **quietistic** turn; at worse, it becomes completely irrelevant. A mantra of 'if we can, we inevitably will' places troubling limits on our critical thinking and moral imagination. We must recognize that the possible – however **captivating**, however **daunting** – is not inevitable.

As human biotech research continues, scientist and layperson alike have the opportunity to deliberate about the ethical **ramifications** of the possible futures opened by scientific research. The science of ethics asks us to justify our actions and account for our intentions. It is not enough just to intend the good or to do something to bring it about. We must give good reasons why we do what we do. In the **realm** of biotechnology, our reasoning needs to address three main areas:

Incentives or the ways that we encourage scientists to do particular kinds of research
Intentions or the goals of that research
Actions or the potential applications of research results

When considering ethical reasons for our actions, it is prudent to avoid "the Dolly effect," that is, attempting to slam the ethical door well after the sheep has **scurried away**. The **unanticipated** arrival of new biotechnologies – from cloning to xenotransplantation – leaves the public, and the scientific community, without a framework for considering the attendant ethical issues. As we quickly learned after Dolly's birth announcement was published in the *New York Times*, paying close attention to the direction biotechnology is headed is infinitely better than potentially overreacting once it gets there. To avoid the Dolly effect, the biotech community must initiate ethical discussions within itself and with the wider public.

Questions Come First

To that end, it is well to begin with some questions. Ethics is about questions: about who asks, what they ask for and how we as individuals and communities respond. In reference to biotechnology, what questions should be posed? What aspects should be considered?

Along with the "golly wow" response to biotech innovation, we must ask, what are the personal and social impacts of biotechnology? What are its potential impacts on our values, our virtues, and our relationships? Does a particular application of biotechnology protect or endanger human or individual rights? Are the benefits and burdens distributed fairly? Does biotechnology advance or **impede** the common good? What are the risks, burdens and benefits? On whom do they fall? How are they distributed? What is an acceptable way to achieve a given benefit? May we do anything, as long as the outcome is good on balance? Or are there limits on what we do, even in the name of human health? And, what – or whom – have we not thought about?

The first step in answering any of those questions is quite difficult for people not well-versed in human biology and genetics: get the facts. Many disagreements result from not grasping the facts of the matter. It is impossible to make sound judgements about the appropriate uses of genetic testing, for example, without understanding some genetic science and the nature of the information gathered through such testing. It is **incumbent** upon scientists and others working in biotechnology to educate the public in general, and the media in particular, about the scientific method and experimental results. The trend toward releasing experimental results to the press before publication in a **peer-reviewed** journal, which is problematic in and of itself, at least requires scientifically **savvy** journalists whose duty is, in turn, to provide an adequate set of facts to the public.

Ethical Reasoning

Of course, facts only describe what is; ethics deals with what ought to be. How do we responsibly move from what is to what ought to be? It is the job of philosophical ethics to provide standards that help us identify what ought to be done.

Utilitarianism: one way to think about "the ought" is through the lens of utility, which looks at various options for action, asking who will be affected and to what extent each **stakeholder** will be benefited or harmed. In the utilitarian view, an ethical action is the one that produces the greatest balance of good over harm or the greatest good for the greatest number of people. Regarding research in human molecular genetics, for example, the utilitarian might argue that the potential benefit of relieving human suffering outweighs the possible dangers of manipulating human genes and evolution through germ-line intervention.

Rights: A different approach presumes that what makes human beings more than mere things is our ability to choose freely what type of lives to lead and the right to have our choices respected. This view from rights describes an ethical action as that which protects people from being used in ways that they do not choose. Importantly, each human has a right not to be treated as means to another's end, even an undeniably good end. The right not to be used encompasses other rights: the right to be told the truth, the right to privacy and the right not to be harmed are among those particularly relevant to biotech research and genetic medicine. For example, respecting rights may set limits on human subject research in molecular genetics by requiring adequate informed consent including an honest assessment of risks and benefits, or it may require that experimental gene transfer therapy to be undertaken only as a last resort. In this view, actions that violate individual or human rights are wrong.

The justice approach to ethics is rooted in the principle of "treating equals equally and unequals unequally." Justice mandates fairness in that people must be treated the same way unless they differ in ethically relevant ways. For example, when two runners cross the finish line at the same time. It is unfair to award the blue ribbon to Jeff and not to Jake unless, for example, Jake has cheated.

The primary form of justice in medicine and medical research is distributive justice, which is concerned with the fair distribution of benefits and burdens across society. Distributive justice, which is concerned with the fair distribution of benefits and burdens across society. Distributive justice seeks clarity regarding those aspects of individuals and society that may justify drawing distinctions in how benefits and burdens are allocated. That is, it seeks to identify under what conditions treating unequals unequally would be justified. Such material conditions could include distribution based on determinations of need, social worth, contribution, or effort. For example, the principle of need would support mechanisms for providing access to cutting-edge treatments to all who would tangibly benefit irrespective of their ability to pay for them. A principle of contribution might suggest that a family who sponsored research into an illness might have more influence on the direction of the research and greater access to its fruits than the rest of us.

The common good rests on a vision of society in which all people join in the pursuit of shared values and aims. Because individual good is **inextricably** woven into the good of the whole community, pursuing the common good includes creating a set of general conditions that are equally to everyone's advantage. Together with respecting individual rights and freedoms, the common good approach requires that common goals, such as human health and well being, be pursued through biotech innovation and a stable health care infrastructure.

A consideration of virtue assumes that certain ideals allow for the full development of our humanity. A person who has **inculcated** these core ideals, or virtues, will do what is right when faced with an ethical choice. Virtues are dispositions that facilitate acting in ways that develop human potential and allow human flourishing. Virtues are good habits in that they are acquired through repetition and practice and, once acquired, they become characteristic of a person. Honesty, integrity, prudence, courage, wisdom and compassion are examples of virtues. Once a person has developed a virtuous character, his or her **inclination** is to act in ways consistent with ethical principles. In much the same way as Barry Bonds is inclined to hit home runs, the virtuous person will be inclined to tell the truth and act with compassion and courage.

Virtue ethics, with the emphasis on character and ideals, captures the idea of "the good scientist" – intelligent, honest, compassionate, determined – much more so than the principle-based approaches of utility, justice and rights. The development of pharmaceuticals for "compassionate use" echoes an ethics of virtue.

Reasoning into Biotech Practice

Those five approaches suggest that biotech ethics should ask five questions:

- What benefits and what harms can be predicted for biotech innovations in both the research and application phases, and which courses of action will result in the best consequences overall? It is important to remember that determining consequences is more or less a guessing game. In instances of profound uncertainty and sizable risk, it is best to **err** on the side of caution when calculating benefits and risks. Neither hopes nor fears should be over-sold.
- Who are the ethically relevant stakeholders, and what rights do they have? Which course of action protects those rights? Is human dignity respected? The consideration of specific individual and group rights requires **coming to grips** with the right to health care – a right that Americans claim but which remains unfulfilled for many.
- Which option treats everyone the same unless there is an ethically justified reason to treat them differently? Biotech justice might hold up "need" as a criterion for access to innovative treatments.
- Which course of action seeks the common good? Certainly, the recent SARS epidemic has heightened concern for the health of the whole and for the creation of common conditions that maximize individual and communal well being.
- Which option best develops virtues? And which virtues, such as trust and compassion, might be particularly relevant to biotech development and human health?

Putting It Together

This framework for ethics does not offer an easy or automatic solution to ethical dilemmas. That is not its goal. The frame work helps identify what ethics requires of us: to consider benefits and burdens, rights and justice, virtues and the common good. Each of these approaches gives us key information about ethical options in a given situation. In the end, each of us brings our moral judgement to bear in carefully considering the facts of the matter and what is right-making and wrong-making about our options for acting. When we do this reasoning together, through public discourse, we have a chance to develop a healthcare vision for our society. Such a vision would provide the necessary – and currently absent – criteria for determining which research **trajectories** to follow and which to ignore.

As we deliberate, we have a further obligation. Because biotech innovations may eventually involve germ-line manipulation, the actions we take today may effect every future generation of human beings, making the coming generations stakeholders in our ethical analysis. Consideration of transgenerational consequences may impose limits on what we do now in the interest of those who come after us. Minimally, we should not knowingly inflict harm. Many indigenous peoples speak of responsibilities that extend to the next seven generations. There is moral wisdom for us in that approach. As we approach cutting-edge issues in biotechnology, this very ancient moral wisdom can serve us well.

Acknowledgements

The general framework for ethical decision making on which this article is based was developed by Manual Velasquez, Claire Andre, Thomas Shanks, and Michael J. Meyer and initially published under the title " Thinking Ethically: A Framework for Moral Decision Making" in Issues in Ethics, a publication of the Markkula Center for Applied Ethics and available online at www.scu.edu/ethics.

Margaret R. McLean, Ph.D. is the Director of Biotechnology and Health Care Ethics at the Markkula Center for Applied Ethics at Santa Clara University.

Jan 1, 2000 Bioethics Resources

1.8.2   General Questions

1. Explain the meaning of "the Dolly effect".
2. Do you agree with the statement of the author that science is political? Give reasons for yes or no.
3. The author mentions problems concerning ethical judgements. Go into detail.
4. Apply the three given points: incentives, intentions and actions to a research field. (An application is for example the research for vaccine).
5. Choose one question from page 81. E.g. What are the personal and social impacts of biotechnology? (An application is for example the research about inherited diseases).
6. Give reasons for non biotechnologists to find an ethical judgement and what does the author suggest what biotechnologists should do to make up the public think about it in a sophisticated way?
7. Exemplify the difference between utilitarianism and rights approach?

1.8.3   Further Research

Make up a presentation in up to five persons about:

1. What is the task of the German Ethics Council? (www.ethikrat.org)
     Draw a conclusion!
2. What is a patent? What are intellectual property rights? Should genes be patented?
3. What are the up-to-date law rules concerning gene technology in Germany?
4. Do a presentation about the EFSA!

1.8.4   Apply the Vocabulary

Fill in the missing words:

1. If you sell more machines in a week, the company grants you _____.
2. This issue is not clear. Cloning is still a very _____ topic.
3. If you write about biotechnology, only very _____ journalists should write about it because it is a very complex topic.

4. If you publish a scientific article, it is given before to a scientist who works in the same field in order to receive an objective judgement. So the article is _____.

5. Sometimes in research, scientists discover _____ results which they have never thought about before.

6. At the beginning it was difficult for him to start a new research project, but now he _____.

7. It takes a very long time to understand this problem, but now he has _____ the issue.

8. Not only consumers are clients of companies, there are many more _____.

9. The first picture of a black hole could _____ its existence.

10. Cloning babies _____ a moral wariness.

1.8.5   Prepositions

Fill in the right prepositions:

1. Are moral values really an issue companies ask _____?
2. I can recommend _____ you this article.
3. Why are you always worried _____ him?
4. He met him _____ Monday _____ 8 o'clock _____ the evening.
5. This article was written _____ Mariam Moratti.
6. Watching TV late at night is the reason _____ his being late to work.
7. I met him first _____ university.
8. He is _____ the hairdresser's.
9. He went _____ the street and then took the bus to reach the station.
10. _____ of the stair was a cat.

1.8.6   End and Beginning of a Word

You start with a sentence that has to do with violet biotechnology. Your neighbor has to continue with the end of the sentence.
   E.g. Moral issues are important in biotechnology.
   Biotechnology for me is a very exciting field of science.
   Science has the duty to be universal.

1.8.7   Create an Ethical Valuable Webpage

Imagine you are the CEO of a biotechnological company producing pharmaceuticals. Write a standard list for ethical values which are valid in your company and published on your homepage. Write about 10 sentences.

1.8.8   Continue the Sentences

Nowadays ethics...
Metha-ethics means...
Applied ethics deals with...
The correlation between biotechnology and ethics...
My conclusion about violet biotechnology is...

1.8.9   Important Vocabulary in the Field of Violet Biotechnology

Noun	Verb	Adjective
habitat – Beheimatung	to comprise – beinhalten	savvy – versiert
ethics – Ethik	to constrain – belegen	ethical – ethisch
disposition – Veranlagung	to advance – voran schreiten	regulatory – behördlich
concern – Sorge	to enflame – entzünden	quiestic – quiestisch
ramification – Verzweigung	to justify – rechtfertigen	troubling – problematisch
reasoning – Beurteilung	to attempt –versuchen	critical – entscheidend
framework – Rahmen	to overact – überreagieren	prudent – vorsichtig
burden – Bürde	to endanger – gefährden	unanticipated – unvorhersehbar
judgement – Beurteilung	to impede – verhindern	well-versed – erfahren
issue – Fragestellung	to concern – betreffen	sound – richtig

1.9   Dark Biotechnology

Dark biotechnology takes the fact into account that biotechnological research could be abused to create pandemics such as ebola.

1.9.1   General Text

Dark Biotechnology and the Laws

Often terrorists are blamed to use biotechnological weapons, e.g. spreading deadly pathogens.

But the point is that states all over the world produce biotechnological weapons although it is against the UN conventions.

In 2001 an anthrax attack was caused by a letter in the USA. Lateron it was proved that the stem of this deadly disease derived from an US laboratory of Dr. Bruce Ivins. It has never been proved how this pathogen escaped from this high-security laboratory.

Till today not much is known about dark biotechnology because it is also not wanted that too much is public about it.

Nowadays triggers for illnesses can be artificially produced in the laboratory to understand their mechanism that is to say that a virus can be created in the laboratory. On the one hand it is good for sciences, on the other hand this knowledge can be abused.

To keep these threats at bay the WHO published a guidance document called: "Responsible life sciences for global health security". Normally sciences aim at improving the health of animals, plants and humans. The document of the WHO would like to inform states and researchers about possible risks including misuse of sciences research and accidents. It proposes measures to minimize risks such as public health surveillance, using ethical platforms, support ethics education and training, boost discussions, make people responsible for their research, train people about new legislation, prevent the access to pathogens in laboratories, implement biorisk management, the willingness of steady improvement and control, using self-assessment questionnaires.

Another guideline is the Biological Weapons Convention of 1972 which came into force in 1975. Every five years the states meet for a control conference. However, there is no treaty about concrete agreements about disarmament.

The convention consists of 15 articles which obligates the signed parties to use no weapons containing microorganisms or any other biological substances or toxins or to store or buy them. They have to destroy all weapons and are not allowed to give it to a third party. In 2018 182 states signed this convention but not every state ratified it.

1.9.2   General Questions

1. Explain the meaning of 'dual-dilemma'?
2. Find out five facts about the WHO!
3. Do you agree that bioterrorism is a real threat for society? Give reasons for or against it!

4. Suggest how to combat bioterrorism.
5. What is your statement about the WHO guidelines and the Biological Weapons Convention of 1972?
6. What means 'to ratify'?

1.9.3 Further Research

Divide the class into four groups. The groups should do a presentation about:

1. Responsible life sciences research for global health security
2. Biological and toxic weapon convention
3. Find out some bioweapons!
4. What can be done to avoid the use of bioweapons?

1.9.4 Crosswords

Find the right words in English. The number of the given letter forms a solution word.

1. Biologische Kriegsführung – _____ 1st letter
2. Impfstoff – _____ 5th letter
3. Krankheitserreger – _____ 5th letter
4. fördern – _____ 7th letter
5. stärken – _____ 8th letter
6. strafbar – _____ 6th letter
7. Richtlinie – _____ 3rd letter
8. bedeutsam – _____ 8th letter
9. wissenschaftlich – _____ 1st letter

Solution word: _____.

1.9.5 German Regulations

Write a summary about the article 314 criminal code (Strafgesetzbuch): intoxication which is dangerous to public safety (gemeingefährliche Vergiftung) in English:
Strafgesetzbuch (StGB)
§ 318 Beschädigung wichtiger Anlagen

(1) Wer Wasserleitungen, Schleusen, Wehre, Deiche, Dämmer oder andere Wasserbauten oder Brücken, Fähren, Wege oder Schutzwehre oder den Bergwerksbetrieb dienende

Vorrichtungen zur Wasserhaltung, zur Wetterführung oder zum Ein- und Ausfahren der Beschäftigten beschädigt oder zerstört und dadurch Leib oder Leben eines anderen Menschen gefährdet, wird mit Freiheitsstrafe von drei Monaten bis zu fünf Jahren bestraft.

(2) Der Versuch ist strafbar.

(3) Verursacht der Täter durch die Tat eine schwere Gesundheitsschädigung eines anderen Menschen oder eine Gesundheitsschädigung einer großen Zahl von Menschen, so ist auf Freiheitsstrafe von einem Jahr bis zu zehn Jahren zu erkennen.

(4) Verursacht der Täter durch die Tat den Tode eines anderen Menschen, so ist die Strafe Freiheitsstrafe nicht unter drei Jahren.

(5) In minder schweren Fällen des Absatzes 3 ist auf Freiheitsstrafe von sechs Monaten bis zu fünf Jahren in minder schweren Fällen des Absatzes 4 auf Freiheitsstrafe von einem Jahr bis zu zehn Jahren zu erkennen.

(6) Wer in den Fällen des Absatzes 1

1. Die Gefahr fahrlässig verursacht oder

2. Fahrlässig handelt und die Gefahr fahrlässig verursacht.

wird mit Freiheitsstrafe bis zu drei Jahren oder mit Geldstrafe bestraft.

Vocabulary	
strafbar	punishable
Anlagen	facilities
Freiheitsstrafe	prison sentence
Geldstrafe	fine
fahrlässig	careless
Leib und Leben	life or physical condition

1.9.6   Describe Anthrax in Your Own Words

Find out five facts about anthrax. Use your own words.

Milzbrand oder Antrhax ist eine Infektionskrankheit, die durch *Bacillus anthraxis*, ein aerobes Stäbchenbakterium, ausgelöst wird. Meistens befällt sie planzenfressende Tiere. Menschen können nur infiziert werden, wenn Milzbrandsporen von Tieren auf den Menschen übertragen werden. Der Erreger ist hochgiftig und kann Jahrhunderte überleben. Deshalb ist der Milzbrand als Biowaffe hoch gefährlich. Es wird in Hautmilzbrand, Lungenmilzbrand und Darmmilzbrand unterschieden. Lungen- und Darmmilzbrand verlaufen häufig tödlich. Beim Tier ist Milzbrand eine anzeigepflichtige Tierseuche und beim Menschen eine meldepflichtige Krankheit. Seit 2003 gibt es einen zugelassenen Impfstoff in Deutschland. 1972 wurde eine Biowaffenkonvention von 143 Staaten unterschrieben, die

die Entwicklung, Herstellung und Lagerung von biologischen Waffen verbietet. Dennoch experimentieren Länder mit Milzbrandbomben.

Vocabulary	
Stäbchen	rod
befallen	to affect
pflanzenfressend	herbivorous
Erreger	pathogen
tödlich	lethal
anzeigepflichtig	notifiable
Tierseuche	epizootic disease

1.9.7   Find the Mistake and Correct It!

In each sentence is a mistake (grammar or spelling).

1. Reliable informations to find on this topic is very difficult.
2. The means to destroy ourselves are the other side of the medal.
3. Its synthesize was a breakthrough.
4. The researchers successful developed a vaccine.
5. He didn't submit the results to the authorities.
6. This knowledge gets more and more important.
7. The result is as important as his ones.
8. This misuse is known to scientists since centuries.
9. Gen modification can also be misused.
10. He is a very carefully scientist.

1.9.8   Diseases Caused by Bioweapons

Find out which diseases are caused by bioweapons or which means are bioweapons or not, give reason for your statement! What are the triggers?*

a) sarin	e) equine encephalitis
b) typhus	f) cereal rust
c) oroya fever	g) arsine
d) rainbow herbicides	

1.9.9   Important Words in the Field of Dark Biotechnology

Noun	Verb	Adjective
biohazard – Biogefährdung	to eradicate – auslöschen	significant – entscheidend
biological weapons – biologische Waffen	to harm – schädigen	clandestine – heimlich
bioterrorism – Bioterrorismus	to pass sth. up – auf etw. verzichten	pandemic – pandemisch
biowarfare – biologische Kriegsführung	to bolster sth. – etw. stützen	toxic – toxisch
toxins – Gifte	to release – frei setzen	unwise – unklug
pathogens – Krankheitserreger	to capitalize – aus etw. Nutzen ziehen	adequate – angemessen
strains – Bakterienstämme	to collaborate – zusammen arbeiten	malevolent – bösartig
rickettsiae – Rickettsien	to anticipate – voraus schauen	ubiquitous – allgegenwärtig
misuse – Mißbrauch	to prevent – verhindern	accountable – haftbar
bioethicists – Bioethiker	to affect – befallen	newfound – neu entdeckt

1.10   Gold Biotechnology – Bioinformatics

Bioinformatics is the use of informatics for biotechnologists to process their data in a quick and understandable why. Statistics and mathematics support bioinformatics. Therefore good knowledge of informatics is an indispensable competence for biotechnological assistants. That is why biotechnological assistants work in a lot of interdisciplinary fields. Nanobiotechnology also comprises gold biotechnology. Nanobiotechnology deals with tiny organisms (10^{-9m}) and materials used for the industry. Biotechnological assistants use large databases to gain further knowledge.

1.10.1 General Text (Tab. 1.11)

Tab. 1.11   Vocabulary for the text: Seasonal Genes

English	German
circadian	Zirkadian (24- Stunden-Rhythmus und dessen Auswirkung auf den Organismus)
to hypothesize	eine Hypothese aufstellen
flu (influenza)	Grippe
assessine	bewertend
PhD	Doctor of Philosophy
inflammation	Entzündung
pro-inflammatory	entzündungsfördernd
biopsy	Biopsie (Eingriff zur Untersuchung eines Gewebes)
pathogens	krankheitserreger
to prone to	neigen zu

Seasonal Genes

This story was originally published by 'The Scientist' on May 12, 2015

   Author: AP Taylor

   Gene expression varies not only during the day but also throughout the year, a study shows.

   Gene expression in human immune cells varies by season according to a study published today (May 12) in Nature Communications – the first of its kind to examine patterns in gene-expression variation throughout the year.

   The results indicate "sort of a molecular signature of the season to humans," said Ghislain Breton, who studies **circadian** rhythm at the University of Texas at Houston, but was not involved in the work.

   In immune cells of the blood the expression of genes that promote information tends to rise in the winter and dip in the summer, the team led by investigators at the University of Cambridge – found. The researchers **hypothesized** that these and other seasonal gene expression pattern may help explain the seasonality of diseases, from infectious maladies like **the flu** to chronic conditions such as heart disease.

   "We now know that all immune cell types have their own circadian clocks, as it is the case for virtually all other organs and cell types in the body," Nicolas Cermakian, who studies circadian rhythm at Douglas Mental Health University Institute and McGill University in Montreal, Canada, told The Scientist in an e-mail. "Moreover, the immune responses, controlled by the circadian clocks, vary according to the time of day," added Cermakian, who was not involved in the work. "What the new study…tells us is that timing information must be taken into account, when **assessine** gene expression and immune-related information, not only in the daily time scale, but also according to the time of year."

   Cambridge's Xaquin Castro Dopico, who earned his **PhD** in the lab of John Todd, was inspired to imitate this analysis after reading how expression of a repressor of **inflammation** in mice, ARNTL., varies throughout the day. At the time, the Todd lab was also collaborating with researchers in Germany on an ongoing study, called BABYDIET, examining the effects of a gluten-free diet during the first year of life on children's development and risk of Type 1 diabetes. BABYDIET requires regular collection of blood from participants over many years. So Castro Dopico used the data to ask "a different question," Todd recalled. "He said, I'll take this unique clinical dataset that we've generated and I'll ask the question: 'Does gene expression change not within a day but across the seasons?'"

   The team began by examining ARNTL expression in the BABYDIET cohort, finding that it had a strong seasonality, with levels rising in the summer and dropping in the winter. The researchers also looked at other clock genes and found that many of them (nine of 16) showed seasonal expression patterns.

The researchers looked beyond clock genes, too. From the BABYDIET dataset, they found that 23 % of all genes examined varied with the seasons.

Grouping the seasonal genes from the BABYDIET cohort into categories, the researchers found that overall, pro-inflammatory gene expression rose in the winter and fell in the summer, following the same general expression pattern as ARNTL.

Next, the researchers turned to publicly available data from two additional studies, on diabetes and asthma, the latter a multi-center study involving participants of summer and winter gene expression observed in the BABYDIET cohort were reversed in the dataset from an Australian asthmatic cohort, indicating that the seasonal trends were consistent even across hemispheres. In an asthmatic cohort from Iceland, which undergoes periods of 24-hour sunlight, seasonal patterns were irregular.

Using genetic markers of each cell type, the team found that levels of individual blood cell types in the BABYDIET cohort seemed to vary by season. Examining the composition of blood donated to Cambridge Bioresource for research throughout the year confirmed that the makeup did vary seasonally.

In a population from The Bambia, a Western African country just north of the equator, the researchers examined patterns of cellular blood composition using data gathered through the Keneba Biobank, finding that the blood's cellular makeup was tied to the rainy season. The researchers hypothesized that these seasonal changes in the cellular composition of blood are the major drivers of the seasonal variation in gene expression.

Studying gene expression in **biopsies** of adipose tissue from an independent twin study also revealed seasonal gene-expression variation, extending this seasonal variation trend beyond blood and immune cells.

An outstanding question is whether expression levels of **pro-inflammatory** genes rise in the winter as an offensive measure against **pathogens** or as a response to heightened pathogen exposure. "That's the 'chicken and egg' argument," said Todd.

Knowledge of seasonal gene expression could potentially help researchers better understand and treat seasonal diseases. For example, it is known that death from cardiovascular disease is more likely in the winter when, according to this research, expression of pro-inflammatory genes is high.

'Our observations help explain why some chronic diseases are seasonal in that our immune systems are heightened to be pro-inflammatory so that when we have a cardiovascular disease, we're more **prone to** developing the pathology that might lead to cardiovascular death,' said Tod. "I'm sure that the greater infectious disease burden that we suffer is also a contributing factor to the changes that we've seen, I think it's both."

Cermakian said it is too soon to consider the clinical utility of these findings. "What is sure," he noted, "is that timing information, circadian but also possibly seasonal/annual, will need to be taken into account more and more in the future, with the aim of providing the most adequate treatment to patients. The response to a treatment might be very different at one time of the year or six months later."

Castro Dopico X et al. (2015) Widespread seasonal gene expression reveals annual differences in human immunity and physiology. Nat Commun. doi:10.1038/ncomms8000

1.10.2 General Questions

1. Give at least three examples how you use the computer for your work as a biotechnological assistant.
2. Give the results of the studies in short in your own words!
3. What might be the further application of this finding in red biotechnology?
4. Find arguments in favour and against categorizing biotechnology in colours. Could you think of any other categorisation?
5. What databases in biotechnology do you use? Give at least one detailed description of one database!

1.10.3 Find the Words in the Text Which Have the Following Meaning

1. In medicine you take a small part of tissue to draw a conclusion for a certain disease.

   _____

2. If you are not 100 % sure about a fact you suppose it might be true and you gather some facts to prove that it is true.

   _____

3. You can divide the year into spring, summer, autumn and winter.

   _____

4. If a scientist works on a certain topic for three years to gain new insights and afterwards he or she can name himself/herself a doctor.

   _____

5. Genes which differ according to time and season.

   _____

1.10.4 Advantages and Disadvantages of Using the Computer Sciences in Biotechnology

Add at least four advantages and disadvantages.

Advantages	Disadvantages
- Evaluating experiments with huge data is easier	- More and more work is done by computers therefore less work remains for biotechnological assistants

1.10.5 Gap Text

Fill in the missing words from the text.

1. If you have a cold, fever and a cough, you have a _____.
2. A _____ is a collection of data.
3. Someone who gives blood to another person is called _____.
4. _____ are the reason for a disease e.g. viruses.
5. An _____ of the tonsils or lungs can lead to a serious disease.

1.10.6 Find the Synonyms and Antonyms

synonyms	antonyms
to investigate	virtual
to collaborate	to be involved
to require	major
to generate	chronic
cohort	utility

1.10.7 Computer Usage for Biotechnology

Give at least three examples of concrete uses as a BIOTA in the field of:

a) office programme
b) data evaluation (excel, auxiliary programmes for the instrumental analytics)
c) process control in the production and development
d) database research

1.10.8 Match the Syllables to Four Words

e.g. = ex -pression, -ercise, -tinction, -amine

1. un-
2. data-
3. re-
4. ir-
5. de-

1.10.9 Important Vocabulary in the Field of Gold Biotechnology

Noun	Verb	Adjective
data acquisition – Datenerwerb	to promote – fördern	circadian – zirkadian
data processing – Datenverarbeitung	to hypothesize – eine Hypothese aufstellen	available – erhältlich
computational biology – computergestützte Biologie	to provide – zur Verfügung stellen	consistent – konsistent
dataset – Datenset	to maintain – aufrecht erhalten	timing – zeitlich
computing – Rechnerkapazität	to install – installieren	seasonal – saisonbedingt
engineering – Technik	to perform – ausüben	cyber – Internet-
EDP – electronic data processing – EDV – elektronische Datenverarbeitung	to process – verarbeiten	prevailing – vorherrschend
implementation – Implementierung	to program – programmieren	promoted – gefördert
maintenance – Aufrechterhaltung	to support – unterstützen	wireless – kabellos
performance – Leistung	to transfer – übertragen	computational – rechnergestützt

1.11   Orange Biotechnology

The topic of orange biotechnology is the reflection about how to teach and what to teach about biotechnology due to the fact that biotechnology is a rather complex field with a lot of interdisciplinary connections. Although biotechnology is a very old science, the word biotechnology was for the first time created in 1919 by Karl Ereky, director of the cattle utilization cooperative who published a book with the title: "Biotechnology of meat, fat and milk production in agricultural large concerns for scientific sophisticated farmers".

Teachers have a great responsibility regarding the viewpoint about biotechnology but also the media. Therefore to think about the consequences not only in teaching sciences but also in teaching other aspects related to it such as ethics is a crucial effect. Scientists, who are teaching biotechnology, have the aim to open the mind of young people for biotechnology and making biotechnology more public and young people interested in their subject.

Therefore pupils should do an evaluation about their perception about how and what they learn in the field of biotechnology in applying different methods to evaluate their experiences.

1.11.1 Application Exercise

Choose a method how to evaluate teaching of biotechnology:

1. Bar chart, pie chart, line chart
2. Questionnaire
3. Scale
4. Target (give every classmate a red dot to attach it on the target)

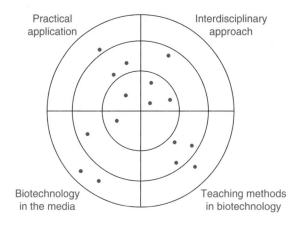

1.11.2 Form 10 Questions in Groups About Five Topics Concerning the Perception of Biotechnology to the Class

It is not allowed to pose a question which can only be answered by yes or no.

1. Do you think that biotechnology has a positive or negative image or both in public? Give reasons for it. (Questionnaire resulting in a pie chart)
2. Do you think that biotechnology is presented in the media enough? Give a number from 1 to 10. (Scale)
3. Are you satisfied with the teaching methods about biotechnology? (Target)

1.11.3 Quiz About Biotechnology

Yellow biotechnology	Brown biotechnology	Violet biotechnology	Dark biotechnology	Golden biotechnology	Orange biotechnoloy
100	100	100	100	100	100
80	80	80	80	80	80
60	60	60	60	60	60
40	40	40	40	40	40
20	20	20	20	20	20

Divide the class into two groups A and B. Each group can choose a field. 100 is the most difficult question. 20 is the easiest question. Who has answered most of the questions correctly has won. The teacher has to ask five questions for every field.

1.12   Bioeconomy

Bioeconomy represents the production of renewable biological resources into value added products such as food or biomass. Bioeconomy wants to reach the transition of the industry by using as less fossil fuels as possible.

1.12.1 General Text (Tab. 1.12)

Tab. 1.12 Vocabulary for the text: bioeconomy: a new model for industry and the economy

English	German
momentum	Schwung
drop-in solution	Einstiegslösung
foothold	Stütze
assessment	Bewertung
mindset	Denkweise

Bioeconomy: A New Model for Industry and the Economy

On the one hand, a bioeconomy relies on renewable resources to meet society's need for food, energy and industrial products. On the other, it emphasises the role of biogenic material flows. The bioeconomy model is expected to reduce our dependency on fossil fuels in the long term. In order to implement the shift from a fossil-based economy to a biobased economy on the regional level, the Baden-Württemberg government launched the Bioeconomy Research Strategy in summer 2013.

It is a very large wheel that natural scientists, engineers, economists, ethicists, politicians and others are starting to turn. A wheel that, understandably, is only slowly gaining **momentum**. After all, it is a question of creating a whole new raw material basis for industry and the economy. It is about developing a new system in which science, industry and value creation interact in different ways than they did before. In the transition from a fossil-based to a biobased economy, oil, natural gas and coal will gradually become less important. These fossil fuels will be replaced by plants, plant residues, biowaste and other biobased materials.

More than ever before industry and science will have to act as a system, and previously non-existent connections will be established between different value creation chains.

Important economic factor: hydrocarbons

The industrialization of the past 250 years is based on good ideas, drive and fossil fuels. Therefore, all industrialised economies are built on oil, gas and coal. Oil plays a particularly important role as it is used to produce organic chemicals, i.e. hydrocarbons. These are the basis for energy carriers such as petrol, diesel fuel and kerosene. Hydrocarbons form the economic basis of the chemical industry.

Solvents, paints, plastics, basic and fine chemicals, additives and many other products are produced from oil using complex, but well structured and established industrial processes. Moreover, our mobility, communication, nutrition, agriculture as well as the energy sector and others are directly dependent on fossil hydrocarbons. Our everyday life is unthinkable without fossil fuels – coal, oil and gas. Hydrocarbons are an important element of the economies of industrial countries where value is created by the efficacy with which hydrocarbons are converted into marketable products; they also make a decisive contribution to shaping the global economic system.

Four challenges

If the vision of a bioeconomy is to become reality, it must not be based on replacing existing infrastructures. Instead a bioeconomy must be built on existing industrial processes. This means that it should initially offer **drop-in solutions** in order to gain a **foothold** in industry. At the same time, new processes, products and value creation chains need to be established. Four challenges need to be solved.

First: The bioeconomy must ensure a solid and reliable raw material base through agricultural and forestry production. These raw materials must be distributed in a way that assures human nutrition as well as taking into account all the economic sectors that use these raw materials.

Waste management is an important source of raw materials in a biobased economy. It can provide large quantities of biogenic waste – plant residues, fermentation residues, organic waste and material from landscape management. These materials can primarily be used for the production of energy, chemicals and materials. However, it will be necessary to adapt waste management material flows to the new value creation chains of the bioeconomy.

The second challenge relates to the conversion of biobased materials into hydrocarbons using so called conversion processes. Conversion processes can be seen as the bridge between petrochemistry and the new green chemistry. The production of hydrocarbons directly from biomass is already possible; however, the methods need to be further developed on a large industrial scale.

Conversion is only one field where a bioeconomy offers sales opportunities. Further potential lies in new materials. The fine-tuned process control of chemical, thermal and biotechnological process steps has the potential to release and use these potentials. One example is the biobased polyamide-5,10 developed by the Biopolymers/Biomaterials cluster.

The third challenge is sustainability. Sustainability is inseparable from bioeconomy. No sustainability, no bioeconomy. This statement underlies further fundamental requirements. Although some have been discussed and dealt with over the past years and decades, they need to occupy a more prominent place in discussions relating to the economy and industry of the future, and include such issues as the effective protection of the climate, water, soil as well as biodiversity. The objective of using raw materials from fields, forests and meadows for industrial production is more than ever associated with the need to manage and maintain the respective ecosystems. This includes rigorous protection of the climate, water, soil and biodiversity. This is where biodiversity research comes into play, which essentially means that the bioeconomy needs to promote a wide range of species, i.e. a biodiversity. It would be contradictory and dangerous for biodiversity if land-use methods that were focused simply on mass production were to be applied.

A bioeconomy also touches on ethical and social issues. Agricultural land is limited. We need to decide how much land is to be set aside for the production of food and feed, fuels and biobased materials. Against a background of hunger, species extinction, environmental and climate protection, the competition between food and fuel calls for a fundamental **assessment** of the respective fields of action in ethical terms. The Baden-Württemberg Bioeconomy Strategy Circle emphasises that the transition to a biobased economy also needs to take social interest into account.

The fourth challenge is to convert technological solutions that are established in the different sectors of the bioeconomy into jobs, production plants, services and goods for export. This fulfills the economic and commercial aspects of a bio-economy. In addition, criteria that enable the economic assessment of environ-mental and climate protection as well as biodiversity need to be developed. A bioeconomy also requires us to change our **mindset**. On the one hand, questions relating to immaterial values must be asked and answered and on the other hand, soft factors such as biodiversity need to be recognized as being able to create ad-ded value.

Bioeconomy research in Baden-Württemberg

These challenges result in a considerable need for research. Scientists in Ba-den-Württemberg are investigating some of the topics that are of key importance in the transition from a fossil-based to a biobased economy.

The University of Hohenheim carries out research into biomass production, bio-mass potentials, land use, land-use changes and many other aspects associated with biobased raw materials. The Institute of Farm Management led by Prof. Dr. Enno Bahrs at the University of Hohenheim is mainly focused on efficiency. How can land be used efficiently? Which plants are best for which purpose? How must material flows and production systems be designed and implemented in order to achieve ideal efficiency?

Prof. Gero Becker from the Institute of Forest Utilisation and Work Science at the University of Freiburg is focused on research to improve the industrial utilisation of forest wood products. His research takes into account biomass quantities and re-sources as well as biomass quality in terms of conversion.

Professor Henning Bockhorn at the Karlsruhe Institute of Technology (KIT) has developed a method known as "biomass steam processing" that enables the produc-tion of biochar from residual biomass.

The transition to a biobased economy cannot be achieved without science and research, i.e. an increase in knowledge. This is why the term "knowledge-based bio-economy (KBBE)" is often used. The Baden-Württemberg government launched the Baden-Württemberg Bioeconomy Research Programme in summer 2013, for which the Baden-Württemberg Ministry of Science, Research and the Arts will provide around 12 million euros between 2014 and 2019. Funding will be provided to re-search that is specifically focused on biogas, the use lignocellulose and the use of microalgae.

1.12.2 General Questions

1. Explain the meaning of biogenic material flow.
2. Give at least three examples of products you use which are made out of fossil fuels. For each example give an idea how they could be replaced by other products.
3. The author emphasizes four challenges. Please explain them more closely with your own words.
4. Which aspects about bioeconomy do universities in Baden-Württemberg research about?
5. Why is biomass not environmentally-friendly?
6. Draw a conclusion about bioeconomy! Give your opinion about the success of bioeconomy.

1.12.3 Do as Much Research About the Pros and Cons Of

a) fossil fuels

   and

b) biomass

   Fill in the advantages and disadvantages into the table:

Fossil fuels	Biomass
Advantages:	Advantages:
Disadvantages:	Disadvantages:

1.12.4 True or False

Try to find out whether the following statements are true or false. If they are false correct the statements.

1. Bioeconomy takes time to be set into practice.
2. Green chemistry deals with the aim to be environmentally friendly and to reduce energy consumption as well as to create very cheap products.
3. A value creation chain includes different entrepreneurial activities such as production of goods, logistics, marketing, sales.
4. The Ministry is funding 12 million Euros for research about "knowledge-based bio-economy" (KBBE).
5. Plastics are completely biodegradable.
6. Cosmetics contain partly oil.
7. Biomass consists out of plant and animal products which are used to generate energy.
8. Waste management has already reached the value creation chain.
9. Sustainability means that the regeneration of natural resources is guaranteed.
10. Prof. Becker does research about the usage of forest wood products.

1.12.5 Explain Three Bioeconomic Products More Closely! Make Up at Least Five Sentences!

E.g.

a) bioplastics
b) sustainable textiles
c) bioactive

(Further information: https://bmbf.de/upload_filestore/pub/Biooekonomie_in_Deutschland_Engl.pdf)

1.12.6 Translate the Following Sentences

Especially with respect to production of medicinal preparations, pharmaceutical companies are increasingly resorting to biological insights. Although chemically produced, medicine still represents the largest share on the German pharma market, so called biopharmaceuticals are increasingly gaining ground. Their sales of 5,5 billion euros are currently 21 % of the market, with a rising trend. These drugs consist of biomolecules that are so large that they cannot be manufactured by man – or only at prohibitive cost. These medications include antibodies against cancer and against auto-immune diseases such as multiple sclerosis, hormones such as insulin for treatment of diabetes and enzymes against metabolic diseases. Techniques from advanced biotechnology developed in the 1980s are applied for their production living microorganisms and cells can thereby be re-programmed as mini-factories (see action "The high-tech tools of bioeconomy").

    Sources: p. 61 in https://bmbf.de/upload_filestore/pub/Biooekonomie_in_Deutschland_Engl. pdf

1.12.7 Do a Presentation About One of the Following Topics

1. Bioeconomy is not only necessary because fossil fuels are running out but also because of other reasons. Give at least four other reasons. Explain them more closely.
2. How could a biobased product be introduced in a company, make up a suggestion concerning
   a) production
   b) sustainability
   c) waste management
   d) marketing

Excursion suggestion: Visit a bio economic company

1.12.8 Insert the Missing Words into the Gap Text

Bioeconomy cares about _____. So for example waste such as paper is reused to remake paper.
The reuse of plastics or glass is part of the _____.
The government _____ all new inventions in the field of bioeconomy.
The products have to be tested in order to know whether they are _____.
Scientists _____ new bioeconomic techniques.
_____ are used for biomass to create energy.
_____ energies are solar energy and wind energy.
Industry and the government have to _____ with each other in order to boost bioeconomy.

1.12.9 Important Words in the Field of Bioeconomy

Noun	Verb	Adjective
material flow – Materialfluss	to come into play – ins Spiel bringen	renewable – erneuerbar
conversion – Umwandlung	to maintain – aufrecht erhalten	biogenic – biogen
sustainability – Nachhaltigkeit	to promote – fördern	biobased – biobasierend
biowaste – Bioabfall	to assess – bewerten	marketable – marktfähig
drop-in solution – vorübergehende Lösung	to convert – umwandeln	decisive – entscheidend
plant residue – Pflanzenrückstand	to investigate – erforschen	residual – rückstand-
waste management – Abfallmanagement	to implement – einsetzen	organic – organisch
value creation chain – Wertschöpfungskette	to provide – zur Verfügung stellen	potential – potentiell
biodiversity – Biodiversität	to adapt – anpassen	effective – effektiv
resources – Resourcen	to interact – interagieren	exctinctive – auslöschend

Bibliography

Bioeconomy: a new model for industry and the economy. https://www.bioekonomie-bw.de/en/artic-les/dossiers/bioeconomy-a-new-model-for-industry-and-the-economy. Copyright BIOPRO Baden-Württemberg GmbH

Chabannes M, Barakate A, Lapierre C, Marita JM, Ralph J, Pean M, Danoun S, Halpin C, Grima-Pettenati J, Boudet AM (2001) Strong decrease in lignin content without significant alteration of plant development is induced by simultaneous down-regulation of cinnamoyl CoA reductase (CCR) and cinnamyl alcohol dehydrogenase (CAD) in tobacco plants. Plant J 28:257–270

Deadly Intelligence: Die Anthrax-Ermittlungen

Evans NG (2011) The good, the bad and the deadly: the dark side of biotechnology. https://thecon-versation//the-good-the-bad-the-deadly

Frazetto G (2003) White biotechnology. EMBO Rep 4:835–837

Gilis J. With an eye on hunger, scientists see promise in genetic tinkering of plants. https://www.nytimes.com/2016/11/18/science/gmo-foods-photosynthesis. Permission: #REF000077117

Hu W, Harding SA, Lung J, Popko JL, Ralph J, Stokke DD, Tsai C, Chiang VL (1999) Repression of lignin biosynthesis promotes cellulose accumulation and growth in transgenic trees. Nat Biotechnol 17:808–812

https://de.wikipedia.org/wiki/Milzbrand Joseph J (2018) Yellow biotechnology application on the food industry through in vitro cell culture meats. https://hopkinsbio.org

Li L, Zhou Y, Cheng X, Sun J, Marita JM, Ralph J, Chiang VL (2003) Combinatorial modification of multiple lignin traits in trees through multigene cotransformation. Proc Natl Acad Sci U S A 100:4939–4944

www.gesundheits-industrie-bw.de/en/article/dossier: Marine biotechnology: unknown sources of hope from depths of the sea. 08.10.2012. Copyright Biopro Baden-Württemberg GmbH.

Matyushenko I et al. (2016) Modern approaches to classification of biotechnology as a part of NBIC-technologies for bioeconomy. Br J Econ Manag Trade 14(4):1–14

McLean MR (2003) Thinking ethically about human biotechnology. https://www.scu.edu/ethics/focus-areas/bioethics/resources/thinking. This article, Ethics 101: A Framework for Thinking Ethically About Human Biotechnology originally appeared in BioProcess International 1(6): 26–29, 2003 and is reprinted here with permission from BP1

Nisria S (2019) Things you need to know about grey biotechnology. www.explorebiotech.com

OECD (2001) The application of biotechnology to industrial sustainability. OECD Publications, Paris

Parkinson's disease vitamin B3 has positive effect on nerve cells. https://www.gesundheitsindus-trie-bw.de/en/article. Copyright – BIOPRO Baden-Württemberg GmbH

Philips T (2019) Bioremediation: using living organisms to clean the environment. www.theba-lance.com

Poirier Y, Dennis DE, Klomparens K, Smerville C (1992) Polyhydroxybutyrate, a biodegradable thermoplastic produced in transgenic plants. Science 256:520–523

Responsible life sciences research for global health security a guidance document. www.who.int/csr/resources/publications

Taylor AP (2015) Seasonal genes. The Scientist 12 May 2015. https://www.the-scientist-com/news-opinions/seasonal-genes

Winkler J (2018) GMO crops could help stem famine and future global conflicts. http://alliancefor-science.cornell.edu/blog/2018/01/gmo-crop-could

www.gesetze-im-internet.de

ZDF infodoku. www.zdf.de

Chemistry

2

Contents

2.1 General Text 1 (Tab. 2.1)

Tab. 2.1 Vocabulary for the text: the importance of chemistry for biotechnological assistants

English	German
to pour	gießen
periodic table	Periodensystem
atomic structure	Atomaufbau
law of mass action	Massenwirkungsgesetz
chemical equilibrium	chemisches Gleichgewicht

Die Originalversion dieses Kapitels wurde korrigiert. Ein Erratum finden Sie unter
https://doi.org/10.1007/978-3-662-60666-7_13

© Springer-Verlag GmbH Deutschland, ein Teil von Springer Nature 2020
U. Steiner, *Fachenglisch für BioTAs und BTAs*,
https://doi.org/10.1007/978-3-662-60666-7_2

The Importance of Chemistry for Biotechnological Assistants

The word chemistry derives from the Arabic word أَلكِيمِياء

There are manifold translations of the word al-chimija such as 'pouring' or 'mixture'.

'Al' is the definitive article in Arabic no matter whether it is feminine or masculine or singular or plural.

First documents can be traced back to 1000 before Christ in Aegypt about chemistry. Chemistry is one of the rare experimental sciences.

It is a common prejudice that alchemists only tried to make gold. They categorized materials, researched metals and developed important chemical apparatuses.

In the 17th century chemistry was divided into pharmacy and chemistry; in the 19th century the industrial chemistry flourished.

The question is why is chemistry so important for biotechnological assistants?

It is important to understand the metabolism of cells which is a chemical process.

Every action of a cell is a chemical process. To understand all these processes a basic understanding about the following topics is necessary.

Periodic table, atomic structure, molecules, **chemical equilibrium, law of mass action**, acids, bases, oxidation, reduction, amino acids, proteins, polysaccharides, fat, lipids.

To exemplify the importance of these topics I have chosen the topic amino acids to show the relationship between chemistry and biotechnological assistants.

Amino acids are organic compounds that contain amine ($-NH_2$) and carboxyl ($-COOH$) with a side group.

Around 500 amino acids are known so far. They play an important role as neurotransmitter and for the biosynthesis that means that plants can synthesize amino acids.

They are the compounds of proteins and also part of antibiotics.

Therefore amino acids play an important role for red biotechnology.

Amino acids have a wide range of application, e.g. you can find them as part of the genetic code (green biotechnology), as nutritional supplements (yellow biotechnology), fertilizers (brown biotechnology) or biodegradable plastics (bioeconomy).

Biotechnological processes cannot be understood without a profound knowledge of chemical reactions including metabolism processes such as the equilibrium of substances. The knowledge about the makeup of atoms is essential to deduce the typical characteristics of the elements and their reactions. The position of the elements in the periodic table reflects their features. If these elements are connected by molecules, new features are created. Finally out of small molecules derive huge macro molecules such as polysaccharides, proteins and nucleic acids.

Biotechnology and industrial microbiology are applied sciences, which have a strong relationship to chemistry.

1.1. General questions:
1. Give at least two applications of chemistry in the field of biotechnology.
2. Choose one amino acid and describe it more closely.*
3. Explain the following words more closely:*
   a) periodic table
   b) atomic structure
   c) law of mass action

2.2   General Text 2

Vocabulary: 1.2 goggles – Schutzbrille

Working in a Biotechnological Laboratory
To respect the safety standards in a laboratory and to ensure sterile work at a work-bench, BIOTAs wear laboratory coats, laboratory gloves and **goggles**. They use all kinds of pipettes such as pistons or glass pipettes. In addition PH measurement devices with accessories such as electrodes, calibration buffer and inorganic and organic che-micals belong to their work. Vibration mixer, ice making machines, photometer, HPLC (high performance liquid chromatography) and GC (gas chromatography) are also in use. BIOTAs use culture media to work with microorganisms, bacteria and fungi to produce cell cultures. Beyond that they use incubators, water bath, gas supply systems, Bunsen burners, laboratory scales and gel electrophoresis. To duplicate DNA they use the PCR. Frequently they use steam autoclaves, nucleic acid sequencer and cen-trifuges.

2.3   General Questions

Name the biotechnological tools of these devices.

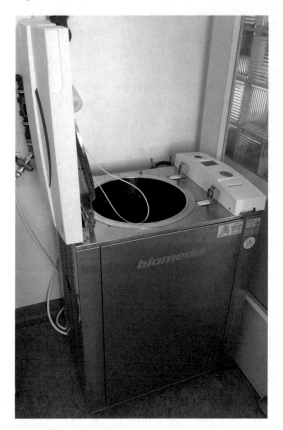

Name of the biotechnological tool: _____

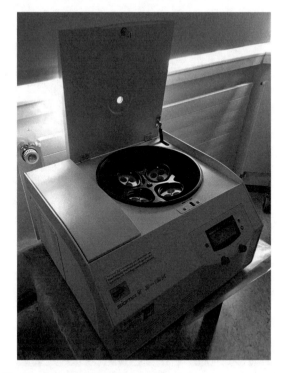

Name of the biotechnological tool: _____

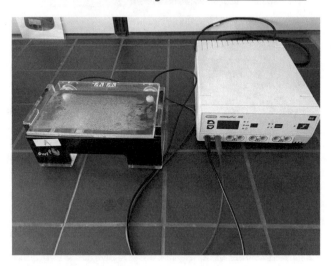

Name of the biotechnological tool: _____

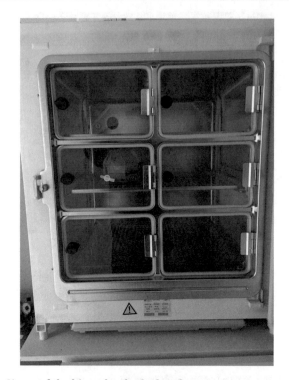

Name of the biotechnological tool: _____

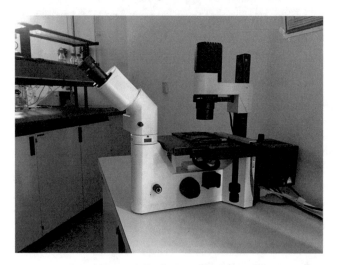

Name of the biotechnological tool: _____

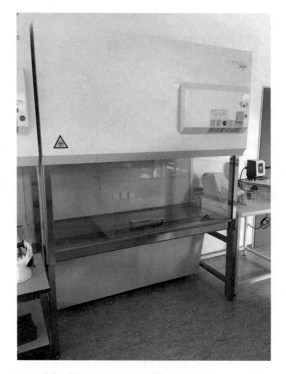

Name of the biotechnological tool: _____

2.4   Divide the Class into Six Groups. Choose One Device

Describe each device and its specific use in detail.*

Tab. 2.2 Vocabulary for describing biotechnological devices

English	German
aboriticide	Abtötung
surgical instruments	Operationsbesteck
chemistry of building materials	Bauchemie
inertia	Trägheit
centrifugal force	Zentrifugalkraft
spindryers	Wäscheschleuder
to magnify	vergrößern
fine and coarse adjustment knob	Fein- und Grobeinstellungsdrehknopf
revolving nosepiece	Drehrevolver
turret	Drehkreuz
light source	Lichtquelle
stage	Objekttisch

(Fortsetzung)

Tab. 2.2   (Fortsetzung)

English	German
slice	Schnitt (der zu untersuchende Gegenstand)
scanning probe microscopes	Rastersondenmikroskope
loosing	entweichen
to vacuum sth.	etw. absaugen
to dispose sth.	etw. entsorgen
exhaust air	Abluft
screw top	Schraubverschluss
manometer	Druckmesser
gas-tight lockable pressure tank	gasdicht verschließbarerer Druckbehälter
bulging	Aufquellen
valve	Ventil
aeration	Belüftung

1. Describe the outer appearance of the device.
2. Explain the function of the device.
3. Elucidate the usage of it.
4. Clarify the reason why it is a biotechnological tool.
5. Exemplify its advantage and disadvantage.
6. Choose your most favourite tool. Justify your reasons.
7. Draw a conclusion!

2.5   Complete the Equations: (Word Equation and Formula Equation):*

$$H_2SO_4 + CuO \longrightarrow$$
$$NaOH + HCl \longrightarrow$$
$$2HNO_3 + ZnCO_3 \longrightarrow$$
$$2HCl + Mg \longrightarrow$$
$$2HCl + CuCO_3 \longrightarrow$$

2.6   Find Out the Cosmetical Ingredients of the Following Cosmetics:* by a Test in the Laboratory

a) lipstick
b) perfume
c) deodorants
d) nail varnish

2.7   Name the Safety Signs:*

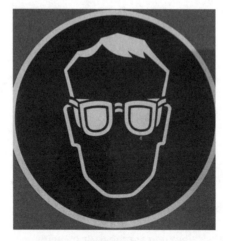

Name of the safety sign: _____

Name of the safety sign: _____

Name of the safety sign: _____

Categorise blue, red, yellow signs concerning their meaning.

2.8   Give a Sample Sentence for Chemical Activities:*

E.g. He analyzed the consistence of the mixture.

a) to distil
b) to dilute
c) to decompose
d) to evaporize

2.9   Tandem Partner:*

See Figs. 2.1 and 2.2

Tandempartner A

Draw the formula structure of the following substances and name the word formula:

1. Ethen – ethene

2. Essigsäure – acetic acid

3. Salpetersäure – nitric acid

4. Sodiumhydroxid – sodium hydroxide

5. Phosphorsäure – phosphoric acid

Solution for partner B

1. Calciumhydroxid $Ca(OH)_2$ - calcium hydroxide

2. Ammonium chlorid NH_4Cl - ammonium hydroxide

3. Schwefelsäure H_2SO_4 - sulphuric acid

4. Ethanol - C_2H_5OH - ethanol

5. Propen - C_3H_6 - propene

Fig. 2.1 Tandempartner A

Tandempartner B

Draw the formula structure of the following substances and draw the word formula:

1. Kalziumhyroxid – calcium hydroxide

2. Ammoniumchlorid – ammoniumchloride

3. Schwefelsäure – sulphuric acid

4. Ethanol – ethanol

5. Propen – propene

Solution for partner A:

1. Ethen - C_2H_4 - ethene

$$
\begin{array}{c}
H \\
\end{array}
\underset{H}{\overset{H}{\diagdown}} C = C \overset{H}{\underset{H}{\diagup}}
$$

2. Essigsäure - H_3C_2OOH - acetic acid

$$
H - \overset{\overset{\displaystyle H}{|}}{\underset{\underset{\displaystyle H}{|}}{C}} - C \overset{\displaystyle O}{\underset{\displaystyle OH}{\diagup}}
$$

3. Salpetersäure - HNO_3 - nitric acid

$$
H - \bar{\underline{O}} - \overset{\oplus}{N} \overset{\overset{\displaystyle \bar{\underline{O}}|^{\ominus}}{\diagup}}{\underset{\displaystyle OI}{\diagdown}}
$$

4. Natriumhydroxid - NaOH sodium hydroxide

$$Na^{\oplus} \; OH^{\ominus}$$

5. Phosphorsäure - H_3PO_4 phosphoric acid

$$
H - \bar{\underline{O}} - \overset{\overset{\displaystyle /O\backslash}{|}}{\underset{\underset{\displaystyle H}{|}}{P}} - \bar{\underline{O}} - H
$$

Fig. 2.2 Tandempartner B

2.10   Complete the Sentences

Chemistry is important for BIOTAs because…

Some important fields of chemistry for BIOTAs are…

Environmental chemistry comprises…

2.11   Important Vocabulary for Chemistry

Noun	Verb	Adjective
agent – Wirkstoff	to distil – destillieren	acidic – säurehaltig
bulk chemicals – Massenprodukte für Chemikalien	to dilute – verdünnen	alkaline – alkalisch
conditions of approval – Genehmigungsvoraussetzung	to decompose – zersetzen	chemical inert – chemisch träge
cosolvent – Lösungsmittelzusatz	to precipitate – niederschlagen	malleable – verformbar
combustion – Verbrennung	to analyse – analysieren	conductive – leitfähig
residue – Rückstand	to synthesize – synthetisieren	saturated – gesättigt
degree of turbity – Trübungserscheinung	to filtrate – filtrieren	volatile – flüchtig
chemical equilibrium – chemisches Gleichgewicht	to extract – extrahieren	gasiform – gasförmig
buoyancy – Auftrieb	to oxidise – oxydieren	homogenous – homogen
contaminent – Schadstoff	to uptake – aufnehmen	immiscible – nicht mischbar

Bibliography

Text written by Ursula Steiner

Microbiology

3

Contents

Microbiology deals with microorganisms such as bacteria, fungi and protozoes.

Microorganisms form the basis of our food chain. They can decompose substances e.g. organic material; they are essential for our food (bred, cheese, wine and beer) and the transformation of substances. On the other hand they can also function as parasites and pathogens. They take part of 70 % of living organisms. Therefore microorganisms belong to the most important part of interest for BIOTAs.

Die Originalversion dieses Kapitels wurde korrigiert. Ein Erratum finden Sie unter https://doi.org/10.1007/978-3-662-60666-7_13

© Springer-Verlag GmbH Deutschland, ein Teil von Springer Nature 2020
U. Steiner, *Fachenglisch für BioTAs und BTAs*,
https://doi.org/10.1007/978-3-662-60666-7_3

3.1   General Text (Tab. 3.1)

Tab. 3.1 Vocabulary for the text: Fungi from Killer to Dinner Companion

English	German
to torture	foltern
to be outraged	empört sein
to be appeased	beschwichtigt werden
spoils	Ausbeute
to contract	schrumpfen
to clog	zusetzen
to wither	verwittern
mold	Schimmel
mildew	Schimmelpilz
rot	Fäule
blight	Mehltau
amut	Schmutz
jock itch	Inguinalmykose (Pilzinfektion in den Leisten)
couch morel	gewöhnlicher Morchel
tallied	zusammen gerechnet
pathogenic	krankheitserregend
benign	gutartig
maggots	Maden
to stipple	tüpfeln
gustatory	Geschmacks-
architectural	architektonisch
wistful	sehnsüchtig
homunucular	zwergenhaft
pincushion	Nadelkissen
to protrude	vorausgehen
hyphal	Zellfäden-
strain	Stamm
mammal	Säugetier
afflicted	behaftet
hibernation torpor	Winterschlafstarre
cusp	Scheitelpunkt
wrath	Zorn

Fungi, From Killer to Dinner Companion

According to Roman legend, there once was a cruel boy who **tortured** a fox by tying straw to its tail and then setting the straw ablaze. The god Robigus was so **outraged** that he punished humanity with wheat rust, a fungal nightmare that leaves crops looking as though they had been burned. For centuries afterward, the Romans sought to **appease** the deity through annual sacrifices of dogs and cows unlucky enough to have rust-colored fur.

Robigus, Lord of Fungus, is still furiously among us, but these days he's collecting his sacrificial **spoils** personally. In the eastern United States, thousands of cave-dwelling bats have died of an aggressive fungal disease called white-nose syndrome, and hundreds of thousands if not millions more are at risk of **contracting** the condition. Frogs and salamanders worldwide are dying in catastrophic numbers, very likely of a fungal disorder called chytridiomycosis, which **clogs** an amphibian's skin and deranges its blood chemistry. Forests along the western and southern coasts of North America are **withering** as a result of fungal blooms injected into the wood by pine-boring beetles.

We have already lost our majestic American chestnut trees to blight and our favorite shade trees to Dutch elm disease. Can't we just break out a few giant bombs of Ajax and wipe the world clean of its infernal fungus, its allergenic **mold** and sporulating **mildew**, its **rot** and **blight**, **smut** and rust, its **jock itch** and athlete's foot that can plague even the most devoted **couch morel**?

We can never rid the world of its fungus, of course, nor would we want to. Fungi represent a kingdom unto themselves, up there in taxonomic sovereignty with the kingdoms Animalia and Plantae, the bacteria and the protists. Some 100,000 species of fungi have been **tallied**, and scientists estimate that at least another 1.5 million remain to be discovered.

Fungi are everywhere, on every continent and in every sea, floating in the air, lacing through the soil, resting on your skin, colonizing mucosal cavities within, and festively decorating that long-neglected peach. And though some fungi are **pathogenic** and will kill the living tissue they have penetrated, the vast majority are **benign**, and many are essential to the life forms around them.

"They are the major decomposers," outdoing even bacteria, worms and **maggots** in their saprophagic industry, said David J. McLaughlin, a mycologist at the University of Minnesota. If you want true antisepsis, look to the fruits of Robigus.

Fungi also have a talent for symbiosis, for establishing cross-kingdom quid pro quos that keep the fungus fed and happy while lending its partner vast new powers. Maybe 90 percent of all land plants depend on the so-called mycorrhizal fungi that **stipple** their roots and feed modestly on their plant sugars to in turn supply them with nutrients from the soil like phosphorus and nitrogen. And botanists suspect that plants might never have made the leap onto land some 500 million years ago without their mycorrhizal assistants.

Fungus may well have given rise to human culture, or at least the comedy of human comity. For a loaf of bread to break with old friends and a jug of wine to help forge new ones, we can thank the fungus Saccharomyces, baker's and brewer's yeast.

More recently, Saccharomyces has served as an agreeable model organism in the laboratory, an excellent way to explore how genes behave and cells, and researchers recently determined that the fungal and animal lineages didn't split from each other until millions of years after both had branched away from the plants.

The defining traits of a fungus are **gustatory** and **architectural**. Whereas animals ingest a meal first and then digest it internally, fungi do the reverse. After latching on to a suitable food source, they release enzymes to break down the substance into a soupy mash of sugars and amino acids, which they can then absorb through the membranes of their filamentous hyphae. Some fungi remain simple, even unicellular, but others can sprout elaborate fruiting bodies packed with billions of microscopic spores, billions of **wistful homuncular** fungi.

The most familiar fruiting bodies are the mushrooms, with their vivid pigments of inscrutable purpose and their still more inscrutable forms – here a swollen pink **pincushion** or a bird's nest filled with eggs, there a **protruding** black tongue or a batch of bright butter coral. Given sufficient food and room, the filaments of a founding fungus may grow over thousands of acres of soil and persist for centuries or millennia, all the while spawning genetically identical mushrooms above ground, and biologists have argued that such **hyphal** masses qualify as some of the largest and most ancient organisms on earth.

Most fungi are adapted to grow in cool or foresty temperatures, maybe 60, 70 degrees Fahrenheit, which is why the pathogens among them tend to prey on plants, or cold-blooded animals like insects, reptiles or amphibians.

Even then, most fungal diseases are not fatal, and the virulent **strain** that is thought to be involved in today's mass amphibian die-offs may have been introduced into natural populations by frogs used in medical research.

With their hot body temperatures, **mammals** and birds suffer from few fungal diseases save those confined to the coolish epidermis. Bats are mammals, but the species now **afflicted** by white-nose syndrome are cave-hibernating bats, and when the bats lapse into their **hibernation torpor**, said David S. Blehert, a microbiologist with the United States Geological Survey's National Wildlife Health Center in Madison, Wis., their core body temperature drops down to just a couple of degrees above cave conditions, as low as 44 degrees.

"This pathogen is treating the bats as if they were forgotten tubs of cottage cheese in the back of the refrigerator," Dr. Blehert said. Moreover, the fungus appears to be unusually virulent. "We're seeing in excess of 90 % mortality at some sites," Dr. Blehert said. Moreover, the fungus appears to be unusually virulent.

Since the disease was first identified west of Albany in March 2007, it has spread to bats in nine states and is on the **cusp** of reaching bat populations that aggregate in groups 300,000 strong, "the largest colonies of hibernating mammals known on the planet," Dr. Blehert said. In an effort to block the pathogen's passage, wildlife authorities are closing off caves to human traffic, for now the only measure they can think of to keep the **wrath** of Robigus at bay.

3.2 Mindmap

Do some brainstorming about

Fungi

3.3 Name the Parts of the Fungus

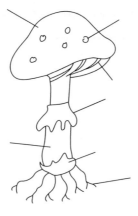

Fungus

spores
scale
gills
stem
cap
volva
mycelium

3.4   Find the Translation for the Parts of a Fungus from Exercise II1.3

Translation:

3.5   What Are Positive and Negative Effects of Fungi?

Positive:
Negative:

3.6   Complete the Sentences

Robigus is…….
The text of the author spreads an atmosphere of……
Five characteristics of fungi are….
Fungi are one of the oldest existing organisms because…..
Virulent means….

3.7 Put the Fungi into the Right Column and Find the German Translation

Edible mushroom	Poisonous mushroom

Cep, led white funneling, chanterelle, fly agaric, death cap, truffle, button mushroom, green finch, boletus, milchling mushroom

Pfifferling, Trüffel, bleiweißer Trichterling, Knollenblätterpilz, Röhrling, Steinpilz, Champignon, Fliegenpilz, Milchlingpilz, Grünling

3.8 Gaptext

Insert the correct words into the text by translating the given words in English:

geschätzt, vielseitig, Hefeteig, Filz, Wirtsorganismen, eukaryotisch, zersetzen, Antibiotikium, Symbiose, wirtschaftlich

Besides animals and plants, mushrooms are the third biggest group of _____ organisms. Fungi can _____ dead organic material. They can also live in _____ with plants or cyanobacteria.

Fungi are also parasites being specialized as _____.

They can cause a highly _____ damage e.g. ergot destroying rye.

It is also said that only fungi made the survival on land for plants possible deriving originally from the sea.

Fungi are used for _____ and the production of alcohol and cheese.

The _____ penicillin is gained by fungi.

Fungi can also be used for _____ to make hats.

Nowadays we know around 100,000 kinds of fungi but it is _____ that there are 2–5 million fungi.

Fungi are very _____.

3.9   Important Vocabulary for Microbiology

Noun	Verb	Adjective
biocatalyst – Biokatalysator	to augment – vermehren	bacterial – bakteriell
count – Zahl	to stain – färben	biocompatible – biokompatibel
yeast – Hefe	to biocatalyze – biokatalysieren	bacillary – stäbchenförmig
barley – Gerste	to afflict – behaften	bactericidal – bakterizid (bakterientötend)
barm – Bierhefe	to lace – einfädeln	pathogenic – krankheitserregend
bacilifocus – Bazillenherd	to colonise – ansiedeln	benign – gutartig
bacterial fission – bakterielle Verschmelzung	to ferment – fermentieren	malignant – bösartig
biocide – Biozid (Schädlingsbekämpfungsmittel)	to latch – einrasten	pandemic – pandemisch
decomposer – Zersetzer	to ingest – Nahrung aufnehmen	airborne – luftübertragen
dyes – Farbstoffe	to digest – verdauen	autotroph – autotroph

Bibliography

Angier N (2009) Fungi, from killer to dinner companion. http://www.nytimes.com/2009/05/26/science/26ang1.html?ref=fungi. Permission # REF000077117

DNA Fingerprinting

4

Contents

DNA is the abbreviation for deoxyribonucleic acid. It involves the hereditary information for humans and other organisms. The DNA is based in the cell nucleus but also in the mitochondria. The chemical bases of the DNA are adenine (A), guanine (G), cytosine (C) and thymine (T). The sequence of these bases is decisive for the make up of organisms. The bases are connected to sugar and phosphate called nucleotide. They are formed to a spiral which is also known as double helix. The fact that DNA can replicate makes life possible. In 1869 Friedrich Miescher isolated DNA for the first time. In 1953 Francis Crick and James Watson presented their double-helix model of DNA based on an x-ray photo of Rosalind Franklin and Raymond Gosling. Francis Crick and James Watson received in 1962 the Nobel Prize in Physiology and Medicine.

Watch the YouTube video:

What is DNA and how does it work?

Link: www.youtube.com/watch?v=zwibgNGe4ay

Summarize the video in your own words (Tab. 4.1).

Die Originalversion dieses Kapitels wurde korrigiert. Ein Erratum finden Sie unter
https://doi.org/10.1007/978-3-662-60666-7_13

© Springer-Verlag GmbH Deutschland, ein Teil von Springer Nature 2020   103
U. Steiner, *Fachenglisch für BioTAs und BTAs*,
https://doi.org/10.1007/978-3-662-60666-7_4

Tab. 4.1 Vocabulary for the text: Curiosity in the genes the DNA fingerprinting story:

English	German
unquenchable	unstillbar
to hybridize	kreuzen
blots	Kleckse
fuzzy	unscharf
eureka	Heureka
seminal	wegweisend
zygosity	Zigosität
to dissect	Aufgliedern
polymorphism	Vielgestaltigkeit
to contest	anfechten
log-jam	Langzeitwirkung
avalancheavalanche	Lawine
to be s.o. hot on the heels	jdm. dicht auf den Fersen sein
modus operandi	Verfahrensweise
exoneration	Entlastung
culprit	Töter
stalemate	Stillstand
perpetrator	Straftäter
mind-boggling	verblüffend
h-index	H-Index
valedictory	abschiednehmend
to slumber	verschlafen
supplanted	ersetzt
beating us over the head	traktieren

4.1 General Text

Curiosity in the Genes: The DNA Fingerprinting Story

It is unusual for a scientific field to be associated with a single individual, but in the case of the subject of thematic series now being launched in *Investigative Genetics*, this is surely so; Alec Jeffreys (Figure 1) is DNA fingerprinting. Having invented the method, he coined the perfect name for it – how different things might have been if it had been called the tandem-repeat-based identification technique (or something similarly dull). He realized its potential and immediately applied, developed and refined it. He then followed his nose to unravel the mystery of the madly mutable minisatellites that make up DNA fingerprints, and eventually to understand the engines of genome variability that reside in recombination hotspots. 'I think I was born a scientist,' he has said (Jeffreys 2005). He certainly seems to have been born with **unquenchable** enthusiasm and curiosity, and it is this quality that has led him on his extraordinary scientific journey.

The story of DNA fingerprinting has been told more than once, but that is because it is such a good tale (its inventor tells it very well himself (Gitscher 2009), and it deserves a brief retelling here. Having noticed the sequence similarity between core elements of tandem repeats in the myoglobin gene and a few other known minisatellites, Alec made a pure repeat probe, and radiolabeled and **hybridized** it to Southern **blots** of restriction-digested DNA. The probe cross-reacted with a set of hypervariable minisatellites, and on the morning of Monday 11 September 1984 the first **fuzzy** DNA fingerprint emerged from the developing tank. In this '**eureka** moment', Alec could immediately see the diversity, and the pattern of inheritance in DNA from a human pedigree. In his seminal paper (Jeffreys et al. 1965) he foresaw roles for the method in linkage analysis, in testing tumour clonality, twin **zygosity** and paternity, in forensic typing, and in **dissecting** fundamental aspects of mutation and recombination processes. In one remarkably productive year these ideas were developed in four further papers (Gill et al. 1985; Hill and Jeffreys 1985; Jeffreys et al. 1985a, b), three of them in *Nature*.

The first DNA fingerprinting application was in parentage testing (Jeffreys et al. 1985a); normally it is the father who is in doubt, but this unusual and challenging case was a maternity test, with paternal DNA unavailable. British nurse Christiana Sarbah's 13-year-old son Andrew was denied re-entry to the United Kingdom after a visit to Ghana, the immigration authorities suspecting that he was not her child. Given three undisputed children for comparison, it was possible to reconstruct the absent father's DNA fingerprint, and to strongly support the claimed maternity over alternative relationships such as aunt-nephew – something that was not achieved with traditional protein **polymorphisms** such as blood groups. In an immigration tribunal, the UK Home Office accepted the DNA evidence, and allowed Andrew to stay with his mother and siblings. It also stated that it would not **contest** future immigration disputes where similar evidence was available, which effectively broke a **long-jam** of such cases, but created an **avalanche** of casework for the Jeffreys lab before the methods were commercialized (Jeffreys et al. 1991a).

Hot on the heels of this came the first application of DNA fingerprinting in forensic identification, in a case that beautifully exemplifies the power of DNA evidence to link crime-scenes, to exclude suspects, and to support convictions. Work with Peter Gill and Dave Werrett had shown that DNA fingerprints could be obtained from old samples, and importantly that the method of differential lysis could yield male-specific information from mixed rape-case samples (Gill et al. 1985). When Leicestershire Police suggested DNA fingerprinting be applied in a local murder investigation it seemed straightforward – two 15-year-old girls had been raped and strangled about 3 years apart with the same **modus operandi**, and a suspect was in custody who had confessed to the second killing. As expected, DNA profiles (now based on specific cloned minisatellites, known as single-locus probes) from semen samples at both crime-scenes showed that the same man was responsible in each case. The surprise, though, was that the suspect matched neither scene – the first DNA-based **exoneration**. A bold police decision then triggered the first DNA-based mass screen to find the true **culprit**. Blood samples were taken from 5,000 local men, and following initial exclusion using protein polymorphisms, the remaining 500 were tested using the new DNA technology. None matched, but the **stalemate** was broken when Ian Kelly, a colleague of the **perpetrator** Colin Pitchfork, told friends that he had been persuaded to provide a blood sample on his workmate's behalf. The eventual DNA profile from Pitchfork himself matched the crime-scenes, he was convicted, and he remains incarcerated today.

As well as human DNA, that first autoradiograph had included samples from various other species, and showed that the core minisatellite probes also detected hypervariable loci in non-human genomes (Jeffreys 2005). Applications promptly followed in mice (Jeffreys et al. 1987), cats and dogs (Jeffreys and Morton 1987), and birds (Burke and Brufod 1987; Wetton et al. 1967). Perhaps the last hurrah of true DNA fingerprinting came with the autoradiograph published to confirm that Dolly the sheep was indeed a clone (Signer et al. 1996). I first encountered Alec when he gave a barn-storming talk to the 1991 International Congress of Human Genetics, in Washington DC. His subject there, described with his trademark enthusiasm, was a near-magical trick that detected and mapped the sequence variation between individual repeat units within a minisatellite, revealing a **mind-boggling** degree of diversity. He had embraced PCR early, showing that profiling could be done from trace amounts of DNA (Jeffreys et al. 1988), and then developing his improbable method – minisatellite-variant-repeat (MVR) PCR (Jeffreys et al. 1991b). With a Y-chromosomal minisatellite in hand (Jobling et al. 1998), I wanted to try it too, and came to Leicester in 1992, finding the same hospitable environment that Alec discovered fifteen years earlier, and, in Alec himself, a generous sponsor. MVR-PCR was perhaps the ultimate DNA fingerprint, but instead of impacting on forensic analysis, it turned out to be a key tool in understanding the complex recombination processes that drive minisatellite diversity (Jeffreys et al. 1994). Forensic DNA testing was moving towards short tandem repeats (STRs), and after using these markers in collaboration with Erika Hagelberg to identify the skeletal remains of a murder victim (Hagelberg et al. 1991), and of Josef Mengele (Jeffreys et al. 1992), Alec's research interests shifted away from forensics. He has, however, maintained his willingness to engage in public debate about forensic genetics and DNA databases.

Alec himself deplores the bean-counting that goes on in judging science these days, but nonetheless it is worth noting that he has well over 200 publications, an **h-index** of 67, and over 21,000 citations of his work, a figure that continues to grow. Since joining the University of Leicester in 1977, he has enhanced the reputation of the place enormously, as can be confirmed by a casual glance at almost any piece of University publicity. It was something of a surprise when he retired in September

2012 since his enthusiasm for experimental science and his continuing technical elan seemed likely to keep him at the bench, pipette in hand, forever. Our Vice-Chancellor, during the **valedictory** address, noted the irreplaceability of Alec, but said that he took some comfort from the fact that 'at least we now have Richard III' (Buckley et al. 2013). The amusement expressed by Alec at being **supplanted** by the skeletal and wormy (Mitchell et al. 2013) remains of a long-dead king can be imagined.

DNA fingerprinting has also, of course, had a massive impact on society. Indeed, it is hard to think of another modern scientist whose work had the societal reach of Alec's. His list of prizes and honorary degrees is almost absurdly long (particularly when set beside those of his departmental colleagues), but it is the public recognition that is particularly telling – Midlander of the Year (1989), Honorary Freeman of the City of Leicester (1993) and Morgan Stanley Greatest Briton (2007). Another honour that many UK celebrities quietly crave is an appearance on BBC Radio 4's long-running programme *Desert Island Discs*. Participants must choose eight records they would take to a desert island and use them to punctuate an interview about their lives, it is said that many a deceased public figure is found to have their disc list stored safely way in preparation for the call. Alec was called (Jeffreys 2007), and his appearance shook middle England out of its **slumber** by including *Feel the Beat*, by Trance DJ 'Darude,' among his chosen records.

As well as a spectacular researcher, Alec has been a highly valued colleague in Leicester – a modest and truly collegiate person who has been a popular teacher of undergraduates, who has shown an almost superhuman ability to unfailingly ask a pertinent question at the end of a seminar (no matter how boring or impenetrable it was), and who has been generous with his advice and support.

These days our universities, institutes and funders spend a lot of time **beating us over the head** with demands for our research strategies, translational research plans, and pathways to impact. As Alec has said (Zagorski 2006), 'If someone had told me in 1980, 'Go away and figure out a way of identifying people with DNA', I would have sat there looking stupid and got nowhere at all.' The story of DNA fingerprinting is a reminder that following your nose and your scientific enthusiasm, can get you a long way.

4.2 General Questions

1. Give examples for the use of DNA fingerprinting.
2. Retell the case of Christiana Sarbah and draw a conclusion.
3. How would you characterize Alec Jeffrey?
4. Choose three songs which you would take on a desert island. Give reasons why and explicitly describe the contents and the musical genre.

4.3   Group Work

1. Choose one reference from 1 to 22 and present it to the class.
2. Present the song: Feel the beat by Trance Darude.
3. Present a portrait of AJ Jeffreys.

4.4   Translation

Translate l. 66–70.
As well as human DNA …

4.5   Vocabulary

Find the right words for the gap text.

1. A scientist has to have a _____ hunger for knowledge otherwise he cannot do his or her work.
2. Alec Jeffrey's work was _____ for the future application.
3. _____ states the reputation of a scientist how often his or her work is cited.
4. The degree of similarity of alleles is called _____.
5. If you cannot recognize something clearly it is _____.

4.6   Plurals

Form the plurals of the following words:

1. bacterium –
2. bacillus –
3. information –
4. mitochondrium –
5. hair –
6. appendix –
7. work bench –
8. laboratory –
9. analysis –
10. synthesis –

4.7   Find the American and the English Expressions for the Following Words

1. Liter =
2. Ausrufezeichen =
3. Klammer =
4. betonen =
5. analysieren =

6. Aluminium =
7. Mais =
8. Note =
9. Postleitzahl =
10. Erdgeschoss =

4.8   Memory – DNA

The memory contains 20 cards. You have to match the cards with another suitable word.
E.g. green biotechnology – GM plants
Make cards with the following words:

DNA – Sir Francis Crick
Chemistry – equation
Microbiology – nucleus
Blue biotechnology – algae
Red biotechnology – vaccines
White biotechnology – enzymes
Grey biotechnology – efficient sewage
Brown biotechnology – droughts
Gold biotechnology – bioinformatics
Violet biotechnology – ethics

Who has the most cards wins.

4.9   Important Vocabulary for DNA

Noun	Verb	Adjective
amplification – Vervielfältigung	to anneal – abkühlen	genetically modified – genverändert
genetically modified organism – GMO – genetisch veränderter Organismus	to alter – verändern	jelly-like – geleeartig
good laboratory practice – GLP – gute Laborpraxis	to inherit – vererben	prenatal – vor der Geburt
good manufacturing practice – GMP – gute Herstellungspraxis	to screen – sieben	affected – betroffen
DNA strands – DNA – Stränge	to locate – lokalisieren	primary – vorrangig

Noun	Verb	Adjective
automated DNA sequencing – automatische DNA – Sequenzierung	to detect – aufdecken	restrictive – einschränkend
additive gene effects – zusätzliche Geneffekte	to soak – aufsaugen	evidential – nachweislich
cDNA - Complementary DNA - zusätzliche DNA	to stain – färben	precedented – vorhersehbar
enhancer – Verstärker	to distinguish – unterscheiden	superior – überlegen
scale up – maßstäbliche Vergrößerung	to apply – anwenden	prospective – zukünftig

Bibliography

Buckley R, Morris M, Appleby J, King T, O'Sullivan D, Faxholl L (2013) The king in the park: new light on the death and burial of Richard III in the Grey Friars church, Leicester, in 1485. Antiquity 87:519–538

Burke T, Brufod MW (1987) DNA fingerprinting in birds. Nature 327:149–152

Gill P, Jeffreys AJ, Werret DJ (1985) Forensic application of DNA 'fingerprints'. Nature 317:818–819

Gitscher J (2009) The eureka moment: an interview with Sir Alec Jeffreys. PLoS Genet 5:e100765

Hagelberg E, Gray IC, Jeffreys AJ (1991) Identification of the skeletal remains of a murder victim by DNA analysis. Nature 352:427–429

Hill AV, Jeffreys AJ (1985) Use of minisatellite DNA probes for determination of twin zygosity at birth. Lancet 2:1394–1395

Jeffreys A (2007) BBC Radio 4: Desert Island discs. http://ww.bbc.co.uk/radio4/features/desert-island-discs/castaqy/0411c084b008fcdz

Jeffreys AJ (2005) Genetic fingerprinting. Nat Med 11:1035–1039

Jeffreys AJ, Morton DB (1987) DNA fingerprinting of dogs and cats. Anim Genet 18:1–15

Jeffreys AJ, Wilson V, Then SL (1965) Hypervariable 'minisatellite' regions in human DNA. Nature 314:67–73

Jeffreys AJ, Brookfield JFY, Semeonoff R (1985a) Positive identification of an immigration test-case using human DNA fingerprints. Nature 317:818–819

Jeffreys AJ, Wilson V, Then SL (1985b) Individual-specific 'fingerprints' of human DNA. Nature 316:76–79

Jeffreys AJ, Wilson V, Kelly R, Taylor BA, Bullfield G (1987) Mouse DNA 'fingerprints': analysis of chromosome localization and germ-line stability of hypervariable loci in recombinant inbred strains. Nucleic Acids Res 15:2823–2836

Jeffreys AJ, Wilson V, Neumann R, Keyle J (1988) Amplification of human minisatellites by the polymerase chain reaction: towards DNA fingerprinting of single cells. Nucleic Acids Res 16:10953–10971

Jeffreys AJ, Turner M, Debenham P (1991a) The efficiency of multilocus DNA fingerprint probes for individualization and establishment of family relationships, determined from extensive case-work. Am J Hum Genet 48:824–840

Jeffreys AJ, McLead A, Tamaki K, Nell DL, Monckton DG (1991b) Minisatellite repeat coding as a digital approach to DNA typing. Nature 354:204–209

Jeffreys AJ, Allen MY, Hagelberg E, Sonnberg A (1992) Identification of the skeletal remains of Josef Megele by DNA analysis. Forensic Sci Int 56:65–76

Jeffreys AJ, Tamaki K, MacLead A, Monckton DG, Neil DL, Armour JAL (1994) Complex gene conversion events in germline mutation at human minisatellites. Nat Genet 6:136–145

Jobling MA (2013) Curiosity in the genes: the DNA fingerprinting story. https://www.investigative-genetics.com/content/4/1/20

Jobling MA, Bouzekri N, Taylor PG (1998) Hypervariable digital DNA codes for human paternal lineages: MVR-PCR at the Y-specific minisatellite, MSY1 (DYF15551). Hum Mol Genet 7:643–653

Mitchell PD, Yeh HY, Applegy J, Buckley R (2013) The intestinal parasites of King Richard III. Lancet 382:–888

Signer EH, Dubrova YE, Jeffreys AJ, Wilde C, Finch LM, Wells M, Peaker M (1996) DNA fingerprinting Dolly. Nature 394:329–330

Wetton JH, Carter RE, Parklin DT (1967) Demographic study of a wild house sparrow population by DNA fingerprinting. Nature 327:147–149

Zagorski N (2006) Profile of Alec J. Jeffreys. Proc Natl Acad Sci U S A 103:8915–8920

Biology

5

Contents

As BIOTAs work with the microscope it is essential to have an understanding of the makeup of the cell which is the basis of life containing the code of DNA (Tab. 5.1).

Tab. 5.1 Vocabulary for the text: the cell – unit of life

English	German
archeans	Archeen
staining techniques	Färbetechniken
specimen	Einzelproben

Die Originalversion dieses Kapitels wurde korrigiert. Ein Erratum finden Sie unter
https://doi.org/10.1007/978-3-662-60666-7_13

© Springer-Verlag GmbH Deutschland, ein Teil von Springer Nature 2020
U. Steiner, *Fachenglisch für BioTAs und BTAs*,
https://doi.org/10.1007/978-3-662-60666-7_5

5.1   General Text

Cell Biology

The cell – unit of life

Cell biology deals with the structure and function of cells. There are several types of cells such as plant cells, animal cells and human cells, muscle cells, blood cells, nerve cells.

A general division of cells is also the categorization of eukaryotes and prokaryotes. Eukaryotes have a nucleus and a lot of compartments whereas prokaryotes have no nucleus. Eukaryotes can be found in plants, animals, humans and fungi.

Most bacteria and **archeans** are prokaryotes. Archeans are unicellular organisms and are mostly extremophiles. Extremophile means that the cells can survive under extreme conditions e.g. in very hot or cold climate.

In the 19th century scientists stared to observe cells e.g. Robert Hooke observed plant-cell walls in cork slices or Antonie van Leeuwenhoek who first described live cells. Other important pioneers are Schleiden, he observed plant cells and Schwann observed animal cells. They defined that all living organisms are made out of cells.

Thanks to **staining techniques** and electron microscopes cells and **specimen** can be described in more detail.

The scientific research in subfields of cell biology cares about cell energy and the biochemical mechanisms which are necessary for metabolism. Other scientists are interested in the phenomenon of the genetic make up of a cell and the transfer of genetic information. Another subfield is concerned with the structure of cell components also called subcellular compartments.

Furthermore an additional interesting field is the messages that cells transport and receive. Last but not least there are scientists who care about the cell cycle.

A new approach which came into existence is the so called systems biology. Systems biology can be seen like the "Russian Babuschka" (little women figures out of wood which are put into a woman figure with a bigger size).

It analyzes living systems in relationship with other systems. This approach makes it possible to answer very complex questions, e.g. the relationship between genes and intracellular processes.

5.2   Questions

1. Give a definition of cell biology! Use your own words.
2. Describe the historical background of cell biology! Use your own words.
3. What is systems biology?

5.3   Name the Parts of the Cell and Match Them to the Picture

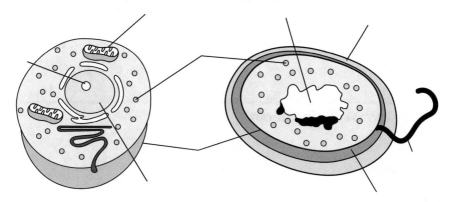

nucleolus
mitochondrium
eukaryote
membrane-enclosed nucleus
ribosomes
prokaryote
nucleoid
capsule
flagellum
cell wall
cell membrane

5.4   Complete the Mindmap

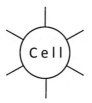

5.5   Choose One Cell and Describe It at Least with Five Sentences

1) muscle cells
2) blood cells
3) nerve cells

5.6   Do a Presentation About

a) Schleiden
b) Van Leeuwenhoek
c) Hooke
d) Schwann

5.7   Quiz About Cells

Two answers out of three answers are correct, odd the incorrect answer out.

1. Humans:
    1. In humans are less bacterial cells than human cells.
    2. have 40 trillion cells.
    3. The majority of human cells are blood cells.
2. Mitochondrium:
    1. has a double membrane and contains the DNA.
    2. is part of procaryotes.
    3. is the reason for diseases in case of dysfunction.
3. Eukaryotes:
    1. have a nucleus.
    2. are smaller than procaryotes.
    3. are only unicellular.
4. Ribosomes:
    1. 2/3 consist out of RNA and 1/3 consist of ribosomal proteins.
    2. were discovered by Albert Claude.
    3. can be found in the nucleus.
5. Flagellum:
    1. is used for the movement of a cell.
    2. is the same for prokaryotes and eukaryotes.
    3. can only be made visible by electron microscopes or dark field microscopes.

6. Nucleoid:
   1. in bacteria also plasmids can be found except nucleoids.
   2. is divided into a base, sugar and phosphoric part.
   3. has no nucleus in an eukaryotic cell.
7. Cell wall:
   1. gives structural support and protection.
   2. In 1665 Robert Hooke invented the name "cell wall".
   3. For humans cell walls are exclusively called extracellular matrix.
8. Membrane:
   1. is permeable.
   2. consists of lipids and proteins.
   3. In aqueous phase its membranes get thinner.
9. Prokaryote:
   1. has no nucleus.
   2. can be divided into bacteria and archaea.
   3. has no ribosomes.
10. Nucleus:
    1. can be found in cytoplasm.
    2. contains the biggest part of genetic material.
    3. mammal cells have no nucleus.

5.8 Complete the Sentences

Cell biology is essential for......
Robert Hooke.......
Staining techniques are used......
Electron microscopes are able....
Subfields of cell biology are....

5.9   Important Words in the Field of Biotechnology

Noun	Verb	Adjective
nucleus – Kern	to stain – färben	intricate – komplex
properties – Eigenschaften	to magnify – vergrößern	unique – einzigartig
release – Freisetzung	to reveal – aufdecken	structural – strukturell
subfield – Untergruppe	to enable – ermöglichen	unicellular – einzellig
cell division – Zellteilung	to divide – teilen	subcellular – subzellulär
intersection – Schnittpunkt	to revolve around – rotieren	permeable – durchlässig
specimen – Einzelprobe	to decipher – entziffern	visible – sichtbar
staining techniques – Färbetechniken	to encourage – ermutigen	initial – anfänglich
mammalian cells – Säugetierzellen	to focus on – sich fokussieren auf	primordial – ursprünglich
slices – Schnitte	to be made out of – gemacht sein aus	extracellular – extrazellulär

Bibliography[1]

Bisceglia N (Hrsg) Cell biology. www.nature.com

----

[1] Text written by Ursula Steiner.

Numbers, Dimensions, Objects, Formulae

6

Contents

Base Factors

Base factors mean that a characteristic feature or action which can be observed in nature is transferred into numbers.

In 1790 l'Académie Française was commissioned by the French National Assembly to introduce a standard system of mass and weights called SI = Système International d'unités. Until today this system is still valid in most countries except in some countries such as the USA, the United Kingdom and Ireland. Also in aviation and the seafaring English measurements are still valid which are different to the SI system. In Germany the Physical-Technical-Federal institution PTB is responsible for the SI system. As BIOTAs have a lot to do with very tiny and very huge numbers, it is important to know the difference between the English system and the SI system.

There was a new regulation about the SI system in May 2019.

There are seven base factors with seven units.

© Springer-Verlag GmbH Deutschland, ein Teil von Springer Nature 2020
U. Steiner, *Fachenglisch für BioTAs und BTAs*,
https://doi.org/10.1007/978-3-662-60666-7_6

Base factor	Symbol	Base unit
length	L	meter (m)
mass	M	kilogram (kg)
time	T	second (s)
electric current	L	ampere (A)
thermodynamic temperature	T	kelvin (K)
luminosity	L	Candela (cd)
amount of substance	N	Mol (mol)

Deviated SI-base factor	Symbol	Denomination
power	N	Newton
electrical tension	V	Volt
electrical resistance	Ω	Ohm
pressure	Pa	Pascal
work, energy	J	Joule

6.1   Simple Calculations and Basic Numbers

$4 \times 2 = 8$ – four times two equals eight
$4 : 2 = 2$ – four divided by two equals two
$4 - 2 = 2$ – four minus two equals two
$4 + 2 = 6$ – four plus two equals six
$1/8 + 1/7 = 1/15$ – one eighth plus one seventh equals one fifteenth
10^{10} = ten to the power of ten

A measurement contains formation of numbers and measurement.

Formula sign $= 1$
Numerical value $= 2$
Unit $= m$
Length $l = 2$ m

6.2   Equations

Word formula and number formula:

$$2H_2O + Ca \quad \rightarrow \quad Ca(OH)_2 + H_2$$

$$water + calcium \quad \rightarrow \quad calcium\,hydroxide + hydrogen$$

6.3   Potency

10^{-6} = micro = m = millionth – Millionstel
10^{-9} = nano = n = part in a billion – Milliardstel

10^{-12} = pico = p = trillions of time – Billionstel
10^{-15} = femto = f = thousand trillions of time – Tausend Billionstel
10^{-16} = atto = a = a trillion time – Trillionstel

10potency	Prefix	Abbreviation
10^{12}	tera	t = trillion of time billionenfach
10^{9}	giga	g = billion times milliardenfach
10^{6}	mega	m = millionfold millionenfach
10^{3}	kilo	k = thousandth = tausendfach
10^{2}	hector	h = hundredfold = hundertfach
10^{1}	deca	da = tenfold = zehnfach
10^{-1}	deci	d = tenth = Zehntel
10^{-2}	centi	c = hundredth = Hundertstel
10^{-3}	milli	m = thousandth = Tausendstel

6.4   Most Important Differences in English and German

1. German: 10,04 m – English: 10.04 m
2. 200.000 m – 200,000 m
3. 1 Milliarde – 1 billion
4. 1 °C – 33,8 Fahrenheit
5. 304,8 mm = 1 foot, 1 yard = 3 feet
6. 25,4 mm = 1 inch
7. 1,60934 km = 1 mile
8. 568,26 ml = 1 pint, 1 quart = 2 pint, 1 gallon = 4 quart, 1 barrel = 36 gallon
9. 0,45359 kg = 1 pound

6.5   Objects

Mathematical objects are numbers, amounts and geometrical figures and bodies.
Geometrical figures are

Dreieck – triangle
Viereck – rectangle
Fünfeck – pentagon
Sechseck – hexagon

Achteck – octagon
Kreis – circle

Bodies

Würfel – dice
Quader – cuboid
Pyramide – pyramid

6.6   General Questions

1. Which measurements do you mostly use in the laboratory?
2. What is the relationship between biotechnology and the given measurements?

6.7   Convert the Following Measurements

1. 3 feet in meter
2. 50 Fahrenheit in °C
3. 23,5 miles in km
4. 0,56 pounds in kg
5. 800 ml in pint

6.8   Describe the Diagrams

Vocabulary for describing diagrammes:

English	German
to increase	ansteigen
to decrease – to decline	fallen
to hit a peak	einen Höhepunkt erreichen
to hit a low	einen Tiefpunkt erreichen
to fluctuate	schwanken
to remain stable	stabil bleiben
to level off	sich einpendeln
to dip	schwach einfallen
to plummet	abstürzen
to raise gradually, constantly, slowly, fast	schrittweise, konstant, langsam, schnell ansteigen
bar chart	Balkendiagramm
line chart	Liniendiagramm
pie chart	Kuchendiagramm
x-axis	x-Achse
y-axis	y-Achse

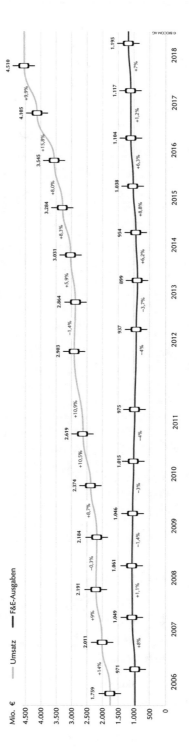

Diagram 1

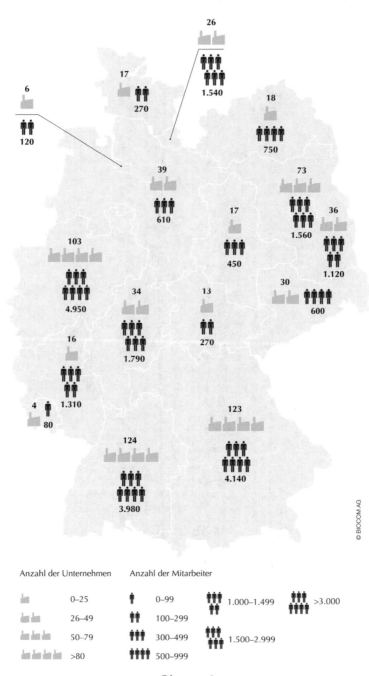

Diagram 2

6.9   Describe the Objects with at Least Six Sentences

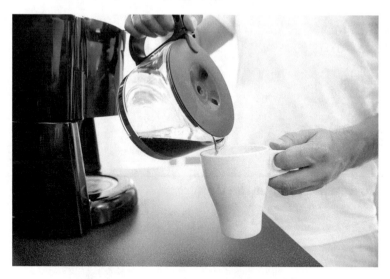

Kaffeemaschine (© ladysuzi/stock.adobe.com)

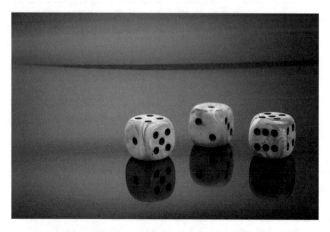

Würfel (© CharlieBfl/Getty Images/iStock)

6.10   Name the Following Calculations

1. $10^5 \times 10^4 = 10^9$
2. $2 + 3 \times (5 - 3) = 8$
3. $4 : 2 - 1 = 1$
4. $\dfrac{1}{4} + \dfrac{1}{4} = \dfrac{1}{2}$
5. $\dfrac{4 + 3 \times (15 - 10)}{10} = \dfrac{19}{10}$

6.11   Do Research About the Unit

a) candela
b) nano
c) ohm
d) mol

6.12   Find the Nouns of the Following Adjectives

a) high
b) wide
c) broad
d) long
e) deep

Bibliography

https://de.wikipedia.org/wiki/Internationales_Einheitssystem
Riech J (2013) Physikalische Gerätekunde. Lernen für die Praxis. Govi, Eschelborn
diagrams: www.biotechnologies.de

Manuals

7

Contents

Manuals play an important role for biotechnological assistants. Mostly they are written in English and therefore a clear understanding of biotechnological devices such as photometers, autoclaves, centrifuges are essential. There are different kinds of manuals: instruction manuals, test records, instruction of use, catalogue offers.

Die Originalversion dieses Kapitels wurde korrigiert. Ein Erratum finden Sie unter
https://doi.org/10.1007/978-3-662-60666-7_13

7.1   Instruction Manuals

Exercise I

Imagine your English superior asks you to tell him what the German manual about the photometer contains. Don't translate the text, write a brief summary about the text in English (Tab. 7.1).

Elektrische Sicherheit

Dieses Gerät wurde überprüft und hat das Werk in **einwandfreiem** technischem Zustand verlassen. Um die sichere und fehlerfreie Bedienung zu erhalten, befolgen Sie die Anweisungen und Empfehlungen dieser Bedienungsanleitung.

Schließen Sie die **Netzleitung** an die Schutzkontakt-**Steckdose** an.

Alle **Peripheriegeräte**, die an das Photometer 5010 angeschlossen werden, müssen die Sicherheitsnorm EN 60950 erfüllen. Beachten Sie vor dem Anschluss die Dokumentation der Peripheriegeräte.

Falls **Abdeckungen** geöffnet oder Teile entfernt werden, die nicht ohne Werkzeug **zugänglich** sind, können **spannungsführende** Komponenenten **bloßgelegt** werden. **Stecker** können ebenfalls **unter Spannung stehen**.

Versuchen Sie nie, ein offenes Gerät, das unter Spannung steht, **zu warten** oder zu reparieren!

Reparaturen am Gerät einschließlich des Austausches der Lithiumbatterie dürfen nur durch autorisiertes Fachpersonal durchgeführt werden. **Unsachgemäße** Reparaturen gefährden den Bediener und führen außerdem zum **Erlöschen** der Garantie.

In allen Zweifelsfällen bezüglich der Sicherheit des Gerätes schalten Sie es aus und verhindern Sie den weiteren Gebrauch.

Tab. 7.1 Vocabulary for the text: "Elektrische Sicherheit"

German	English
einwandfrei	impeccable
Netzleitung	power line
Steckdose	plug socket
Peripheriegeräte	peripheral devices
Abdeckungen	caps
zugänglich	accessible
spannungsführend	to be energised
etw. bloss legen	to lay sth. bare
Stecker	plug
unter Spannung stehen	to be energised
warten	to service
inappropriately (adv.)	unsachgemäß
Erlöschen	expiry

7.2   Test Records

The polymerase chain reaction is one of the activities for the BIOTAs which are very important. It enables to replicate the hereditary substance DNS in vitro. PCR is used to recognise hereditary diseases and virus infections. It is also applied for the recognition of genetic fingerprints and for cloning of genes as well as for ancestry expertise. In 1983 Kary Mullis developed the PCR and he was awarded in 1993 the Nobel Prize for Chemistry.

In the following you find a test record (however abbreviated) for PCR.

Lesson 1 – Cheek Cell DNA Template Preparation (Lab Protocol)
1. Each member of your team should have 1 **screwcap tube** containing 200 µl InstaGene™ matrix, 1.5 ml micro test tube, and a cup containing 10 ml of 0.9 % saline solution. Label one of each tube and a cup with your initials.
2. Do not throw away the saline after completing this step. Pour the saline from the cup into your mouth. **Rinse** vigorously for 30 seconds. Expel the saline back into the cup.
3. Set a P-1,000 µl micropipet to 1,000 µl and transfer 1 ml of your oral rinse into the micro test tube with your initials. If no P-1,000 µl is available, carefully pour – 1 ml of your **swished** saline into the micro test tube (use the markings on the side of the micro test tube to estimate 1 ml).
4. **Spin** your tube in a balanced centrifuge for 2 minutes at full speed. When the centrifuge has completely stopped, remove your tube. You should be able to see a **pellet** of **whitish** cells at the bottom of the tube. Ideally, the pellet should be about the size of a match head. If you can't see your pellet, or your pellet is too small, **pour off** the saline **supernatant**, add more of your saline rinse, and spin again.
5. Pour off the supernatant and **discard**. Taking care not to lose your cell pellet, carefully **blot** your micro test tube on a tissue or paper towel. It's ok for a small amount of saline (~50 µl about the same size as your pellet) to remain in the bottom of the tube.
6. **Resuspend** the pellet thoroughly by vortexing or flicking the tubes until no cell clumps remain.
7. Using an adjustable volume micropipet set to 20 µl, transfer your resuspended cells into the screwcap tube containing the InstaGene with your initials. You may need to use the pipet a few times to transfer all of your cells.
8. Screw the caps tightly on the tubes. Shake or vortex to mix the contents.
9. Place the tubes in the foam micro test-tube holder. When all members of your team have collected their samples, **float** the holder with tubes in a 56 °C water bath for 10 minutes. At the halfway point (5 minutes), shake or vortex the tubes several times. Place the tubes back in the water bath for the remaining 5 minutes.
10. Remove the tubes from the water bath and shake them several times. Now float the holder with tubes in a 100 °C water bath for 5 minutes.

Tab. 7.2 Vocabulary for the text: Lesson 1: Cheek Cell DNA Template Preparation (Lab Protocol)

English	German
screwcap tube	Röhrchen mit Schraubverschluss
to rinse	ausspülen
swished	durchgelaufen
to spin	drehen
pellet	Kügelchen
whitish	weißlich
to pour sth. off	etw. abgießen
supernatant	überstehend, Überschüssiges
to discard	ausschalten
to blot	kleksen
to resuspend	resuspendieren
to float	gleiten

11. Remove the tubes from the 100 °C water bath and shake or vortex several times to resuspend the sample. Place the eight tubes in a balanced arrangement in a centrifuge. Pellet the matrix by spinning for 5 minutes at $6{,}000 \times g$ (or 10 minutes at $2{,}000 \times g$).

12. Store your screwcap tube in the refrigerator until the next laboratory period, or proceed to step 2 of lesson 2 if your teacher instructs you to do so (Tab. 7.2).

Lesson 2 PCR Amplification (Lab Protocol)

1. Obtain your screwcap tube that contains your genomic DNA **template** from the refrigerator. Centrifuge your tubes for 2 minutes at $6000 \times g$ or for 5 minutes at $2000 \times g$ in a centrifuge.

2. Each member of the team should obtain a PCR tube and capless micro test tube. **Label** each PCR tube on the side of the tube with your initials and place the PCR tube into the capless micro test tube as shown. Place the PCR tube in the **foam** micro test tube holder.

3. Transfer 20 µl of your DNA template from the supernatant in your screwcap tube into the bottom of the PCR tube. Do not transfer any of the matrix **beads** into the PCR reaction because they will **inhibit** the PCR reaction.

4. Locate the tube of yellow PCR master mix (labeled "Master") in your ice bucket. Transfer 20 µl of the master mix into your PCR tube. Mix by pipetting up and down 2–3 times. Cap the PCR tube lightly and keep it on ice until instructed to proceed to the next step. Avoid **bubbles**, especially in the bottom of the tubes.

5. Remove your PCR tube from the capless micro test tube and place the tube in the Gene Cycler or MyCycler thermal cycler.

6. When all of the PCR samples are in the thermal cycler, the teacher will begin the PCR reaction. The reaction will undergo 40 cycles of amplification, which will take approximately 3 hours.

7. If your teacher instructs you to do so, you will now pour your agarose gels (the gels may have been prepared ahead of time by the teacher).

Tab. 7.3 Vocabulary for the
text: Lesson 2: PCR Amplification (Lab Protocol)

English	German
template	Vorlage
to label	beschriften
foam	Schaum
beads	Tropfen
to inhibit	verhindern
bubbles	Blasen
pre-denaturation	Vorvergällung
to denature	vergällen
to anneal	abkühlen

Program Gene Cycler or MyCycler thermal cycler.

The thermal cycler should be programmed for 3 steps in cycle 2, which will repeat 40 times. The final cycle 3 ensures that the final extension reaction goes to completion and all possible PCR products are made. The PCR reaction will take approximately 3.5 hours (Tab. 7.3).

Cycle	Step	Function	Temperature	Time
1	Step 1	**Pre-denaturation**	94 °C	2 minutes
	Repeat 1 time			
2	Step 1	**Denature**	94 °C	1 minute
	Step 2	**Anneal**	60 °C	1 minute
	Step 3	Extend	72 °C	2 minutes
	Repeat 40 times			
3	Step 1	Final extension	72 °C	10 minutes
	Repeat 1 time			

Refer to the Gene Cycler or MyCycler instruction manual for specific programming instructions or to the instructions in Appendix H.

Lesson 3: Gel Electrophoresis of Amplified PCR Samples (Lab Protocol)
1. Remove your PCR samples from the **thermal cycler** and place it in the micro test tube holder. If a centrifuge is available, place the PCR tubes in the capless micro test tubes and pulse-spin the tubes (~3 seconds at $2000 \times g$) to bring the condensation that formed on the **lids** to the bottom of the tubes.
2. Add 10 µl of PV92 XC loading dye to each PCR tube and mix gently.
3. Obtain an agarose gel (either the one you poured or one pre-poured by your teacher). Place the **casting tray** with the **solidified** gel in it, onto the platform in the gel box. The wells should be at the cathode (−) end of the box, where the black lead is connected. Very carefully remove the **comb** from the gel by pulling it straight up, slowly.
4. Pour −275 ml of electrophoresis buffer into the electrophoresis chamber, until it just covers the **wells.**
5. Using a clean tip for each sample, load the samples into the 8 wells of the gel in the following order:

Lane	Sample	Load volume
1	NMR (DNA standard)	10 µl
2	Homozygous (+/+) control	10 µl
3	Homozygous (−/−) control	10 µl
4	Heterozygous (+/−) control	10 µl
5	Student 1	20 µl
6	Student 2	20 µl
7	Student 3	20 µl
8	Student 4	20 µl

6. Secure the lid on the gel box. The lid will attach to the base in only one orientation red to red and black to black. Connect the electrical **leads** to the power supply.
7. Turn on the power supply. Set it to 100 V and electrophorese the samples for 30 minutes.
8. When electrophoresis is complete, turn off the power and remove the lid from the gel box. Carefully remove the gel tray and the gel from the gel box. Be careful, the gel is very slippery. **Nudge** the gel off the gel tray with your thumb and carefully slide it into your plastic staining tray (Tab. 7.4).

Staining of Agarose Gels

The moment of truth has arrived. What is your genotype? Are you a homozygote or a heterozygote? To find out, you will have to stain your agarose gel. Since DNA is naturally colorless, it is not immediately visible in the gel. **Unaided visual examination** of gel after electrophoresis indicates only the positions of the loading dyes and not the positions of the DNA fragments. DNA fragments are visualized by staining the gel with a blue dye called Fast Blast DNA stain. These blue dye molecules strongly bind to the DNA frag-

Tab. 7.4 Vocabulary for the text: Lesson 3: Gel Electrophoresis of Amplified PCR Samples (Lab Protocol)

English	German
thermal cycler	Thermocycler
lids	Deckel
casting tray	Gießschale
to solidify	verfestigen
comb	Kamm
wells	Wasserbehälter
leads	Kabel
to nudge	anstoßen
unaided visual examination	Sichtprüfung ohne optische Vergrößerung
blast	explodierende
to notch	einkerben
noncarcinogenic	nicht krebserregend

ments and allow DNA to become visible. These visible bands of DNA may then be traced, photographed, sketched or retained as a permanently dried gel for analysis.

Directions for Using Fast Blast DNA Stain

Below are two protocols for using fast **blast** DNA stain in the classroom. Use protocol for quick staining of gels to visualize DNA bands in 12–15 minutes, and protocol 2 for overnight staining. Depending on the amount of time available, your teacher will decide which protocol to use. Two student teams will stain the gels per staining tray (you may want to **notch** gel corners for identification). Mark staining trays with initials and class period before beginning this activity.

WARNING

Although fast blast DNA stain is nontoxic and **noncarcinogenic**, latex or vinyl gloves should be worn while handling the stain or stained gels to keep hands from becoming stained blue. Lab coats or other protective clothing should be worn to avoid staining clothes.

Lesson 4: Analysis and Interpretation of Results

Remember that his Alu sequence is inserted into a noncoding region of the PV92 locus on chromosome 16 and is not related to a particular disease, nor does it code for any protein sequence that can be used to study human genotypic frequencies (Tab. 7.5).

Because Alu repeats appear in the general population **at random**, the Alu insert in chromosome 16 is very useful for the study of gene frequencies in localized human populations. Theoretically, in some small, geographically isolated populations, all individuals may be homozygous +/+. In others, the individuals may all be homozygous −/− in a "melting-pot" population, the three genotypes (+/+, +/−. −/−) may exist in equilibrium.

The frequencies of genotypes and alleles are basic characteristics that population geneticists use to describe and analyze populations. The results you obtain in this exercise provide a real-life opportunity to calculate genotypic and allelic frequencies of the Alu insert in your class and to use the Hardy-Weinberg equation.

The results of the PCR reactions reveal your and your classmates genotypes: +/+, +/−, and −/−. Knowing your genotypes, you can **count up** the alleles of your class 'population' and determine their frequencies. You can then compare the allelic and genotypic frequencies of your class population to published reports of larger population sizes.

Tab. 7.5 Vocabulary for the text Lesson 4: Analysis and Interpretation of Results

English	German
at random	zufällig
count sth. up	etw. zusammen rechnen
respectively	entsprechend
Hardy-Weinberg equation	Hardy-Weinberg-Gleichung geht auf den Arzt Hardy und den Vererbungsforscher Weinberg zurück, um anhand von einer Gleichung die Populationsgenetik berechnen zu können.

Focus Questions
1. What is your genotype for the Alu insert in your PV92 region?
2. What are the genotypic frequencies of +/+, +/−, and −/− in your class population? Fill in the table below with your class data. (Tab. 1, p. 135)

Allelic frequencies can be calculated from the numbers and frequencies of the genotypes in the population. Population geneticists use the terms p and q to represent the frequencies of the (+) and (−) alleles, **respectively**. Allele frequencies can be calculated from either the numbers or the frequencies of the genotypes (since they are related to each other).

$$p = \text{frequency of } (+) \text{ allele} =$$

$$\frac{\text{number of } (+) \text{ alleles}}{\text{total number of alleles } (\text{both} + \text{and} -)}$$

$$\frac{2 \left(\# \text{ of } +/+ \text{ students} \right) + 1 \left(\# \text{ of } +/- \text{ students} \right)}{\text{total number of alleles } (\text{both} + \text{and} -)}$$

$$\text{frequency of } (+/+) \text{ students} + \tfrac{1}{2} \left(\text{frequency of } (+/-) \text{ students} \right)$$

$$q = \text{frequency of } (-) \text{ allele} =$$

$$\frac{\text{number of } (-) \text{ alleles}}{\text{total number of alleles } (\text{both} + \text{and} -)}$$

$$\frac{2 \left(\# \text{ of } -/- \text{ students} \right) + 1 \left(\# \text{ of } +/- \text{ students} \right)}{\text{total number of alleles } (\text{both} + \text{and} -)}$$

$$\text{frequency of } (-/-) \text{ students} + \tfrac{1}{2} \left(\text{frequency of } (+/-) \text{ students} \right)$$

3. What is the frequency of each allele in your class sample? Fill in the table below with your class data. Remember, a class of 32 students (N) will have a total of 64 (2N) instances of each locus. (Tab. 2, p. 135)
4. The following table presents data from a USA-wide random population study. (Tab. 3, p. 136)

Now, using the date above, calculate the allelic frequencies for the USA data as you did for your class population in Tab. 2. (Tab. 2, p. 135)

5. How do your actual class data for genotypic and allelic frequencies compare with those of the random sampling of the USA population? Would you expect them to match? What reasons can you think of to explain the differences or similarities?
   The **Hardy-Weinberg equation**, $p^2 + 2pq + q^2 = 1$, is one of the foundations of population genetics. It is the algebraic expansion of $(p + q)^2 = 1$, where $p + q = 1$. The equation describes the frequencies of genotypes in a population that is at "genetic equilibrium", meaning that the frequencies are stable from generation to generation. The Hardy-Weinberg theory states that, for a population to achieve this equilibrium, the population must be quite large, the members

must make randomly and produce offspring with equal success, and then must be no migration of individuals into or out of the population, or an excessive mutation converting one allele to another. Given these conditions, and the allelic frequencies p and q, the Hardy-Weinberg equation says that

$$\mathbf{P^2} = \textbf{the expected frequency of the} \left(+/+\right) \textbf{genotype in the population}$$
$$\mathbf{2pq} = \textbf{the expected frequency of the} \left(+/-\right) \textbf{genotype in the population}$$
$$\mathbf{q^2} = \textbf{the expected frequency of the} \left(-/-\right) \textbf{genotype in the population}$$

It is important to understand that p^2, $2pq$, and q^2 are expected, theoretical genotype frequencies of a population under Hardy-Weinberg equilibrium conditions, and they may not be realized in real-life population samples if one of the conditions is not that. These theoretical frequencies are calculated using the observed values for p and q they may not be the same as the observed genotypic frequencies such as those shown in Tab. 1. If the observed and expected genotypic frequencies are the same, this indicates that the population is in Hardy-Weinberg genetic equilibrium.

6. Using the values for p and q that you calculated in Tab. 2 for your class population, calculate p^2, $2\ pq$ and q^2. Do they come out to be the same as the genotype frequencies that you found in Tab. 1?

    If they do, your class resembles a Hardy-Weinberg genetic equilibrium. If you observed (actual) genotype frequencies are not the same as the expected values, what might be some of the reasons for the difference?

7. Using the values for p and q that you calculated in Tab. 4 for the USA population sample, calculate p^2, $2pq$, and q^2. Do they come out to be the same as the genotype frequencies that you found in Tab. 3? Does the USA-wide sample suggest that the population of the USA is in Handy-Weinberg equilibrium?

Lesson 5 Analysis of Classroom Data Using Bioinformatics
Bioinformatics is a discipline that integrates mathematical, statistical, and computer tools to collect and process biological data. Bioinformatics has become an important tool in

Tab. 1 Observed genotype frequencies for the class

Category	Number	Frequency (# of genotypes/total)
Homozygous (+/+)		
Heterozygous (+/−)		
Homozygous (−/−)		
	Total =	= 1.00

Tab. 2 Calculated allelic frequencies for the class

Category	Number	Frequency
(+) alleles		p =
(−) alleles		q =
	Total alleles =	= 1.00

Tab. 3 Genotypic frequencies for Alu in a USA Sample

Category	Number	Frequency
Homozygous (+/+)	2422	0.24
Heterozygous (+/−)	5528	0.55
Homozygous (−/−)	2050	0.21
	Total = 10,000	= 1.00

Tab. 4 Calculated allelic
frequencies for USA

Category	Number	Frequency
(+) alleles		p =
(−) alleles		q =
	Total alleles =	= 1.00

recent years for analyzing the extraordinary large amount of biological information that is being generated by researchers around the world. In Lesson 5, you will perform a bio-informatics exercise to investigate the genotypic frequencies for the Alu polymorphism in your class population and compare them with the genotypic frequencies of other populations.

Following PCR amplification and electrophoresis of your samples, you will analyze your experimental data to determine your genotypes for the Alu insertion within the PV92 locus on chromosome 16. The classroom genotype data can then be entered into the Allele Server database located at Cold Spring Harbor Laboratory's Dolan DNA Learning Center. Allele Server is a Web-based database that contains genotype data from a range of populations around the world as well as other classrooms and teacher training workshops. It also provides a collection of statistical analysis tools to examine the Alu insertion polymorphism at the population level. You can either analyze your classroom data as an individual population or compare your population with other populations in the database.

Once you enter classroom data into Allele Server, you can perform a Chi-square analysis to compare the Alu genotype frequencies within the class population with those predicted by the Hardy-Weinberg equation. The genotypic frequencies of the class population can also be compared with the genotypic frequencies of another population in the database, using the Chi-square analysis.

Using Allele Server
Note: The Dolan DNA Learning Center website is continually updated. Some of the following information may change.

1. On your Web browser, go to vector.cshl.org
2. Log in to Allele Server using the username and password your instructor provides.
3. Once you have logged in, follow instructions provided in the pop-up window for using Allele Server. You may also open a new window and go to dnalc.org/help/sad/topic_3.html to get more detailed instructions. Follow the detailed instructions on how to populate the workspace, analyze groups, compare groups, and query the database.

Remember that as a registered user, you may store any groups that you loaded in your personal Allele Server database and analyze them at your convenience.

7.3 Exercises

7.3.1 General Questions

1. Summarise the lessons 1–5 in brief.
2. Describe the usage and the importance of the PCR.*
3. Clarify the meaning of the Hardy-Weinberg equation!*
4. Define the use of allele more closely!*
5. If you compare the use of language for manuals and other texts what is the difference?

7.3.2 Gap Text

Fill in the right words:

1. The centrifuge _____ around its own axis.
2. Don't forget to _____ your devices in the laboratory if you have finished your work.
3. A special gel is used to _____ it into _____.
4. The gel is not liquid it _____ over time.
5. If you let apples lie around for too long they _____.

7.3.3 Write Your Own Manual

Choose a biotechnological process and write your own manual. Do this task in pairs.*

7.3.4 Instruction for Use

Centrifuges
Centrifuges are used in the laboratory to separate substances such as suspensions, emulsions and gas mixtures due to their different density, inertia and on the basis of the centrifugal force (Tab. 7.6).

Tab. 7.6 Vocabulary for the text: Bedienung und Inbetriebnahme einer Zentrifuge

German	English
Inbetriebnahme	startup
anschließen	to connect
Netzkabel	power cable
dazugehörig	corresponding
ausbalancieren	to balance
Laufzeit	runtime
ablaufen	to run off
Riegel	lock
Stillstand	stagnancy
abbremsen	to slow sth. down
zentrifugieren	to centrifuge
Tarierung	taring
Antrieb	power unit
schonen	to preserve
Gehäuse	box

Bedienung: Inbetriebnahme

- **Schließen** Sie das **Netzkabel an** und stellen Sie den Netzschalter auf die Position „I".
- Öffnen Sie den Deckel und beladen Sie den **dazugehörigen** Rotor mit den Proben.
- Stellen Sie sicher, dass die Proben **ausbalanciert** sind. (Lesen Sie dazu den folgenden Abschnitt „Beladen des Rotors".)
- Schließen Sie den Deckel. Der Rotor beschleunigt dann schnell auf die maximale Geschwindigkeit von 5500 rpm.
- Wenn die gewünschte **Laufzeit abgelaufen** ist, drücken Sie auf den Deckel**riegel**, um die Zentrifuge zu öffnen. Der Rotor wird nun rasch bis zum **Stillstand abgebremst** und die Proben können dann entnommen werden.

ACHTUNG: Fassen Sie niemals mit den Händen in den Rotorbereich, bevor dieser nicht vollkommen still steht.

ACHTUNG:

Zentrifugieren Sie niemals mit Rotoren, die bereits deutliche Korrosionsspuren oder mechanische Schäden aufweisen.

Zentrifugieren Sie niemals mit stark korodierenden Substanzen, die Materialschäden versursachen und die mechanische Festigkeit von Rotoren und Zentrifuge beeinträchtigen können.

Beladen des Rotors

Die Rotoren dürfen nur symmetrisch beladen werden (siehe Anhang 1). Die Adapter dürfen nur mit den dafür vorgesehenen Gefäßen beladen werden. Die Gewichtsunterschiede zwischen den gefüllten Probengefäßen sind gering zu halten, dazu wird die **Tarierung** mit einer Waage empfohlen. Dadurch wird der **Antrieb geschont** und die Laufgeräusche verringert.

Der Netzschalter ist hinten links an der Rückwand des **Gehäuses**.

Exercise

Imagine you have a new colleague from GB and you should explain her how the centrifuge works. Don't translate the text. Explain how to handle a centrifuge.

What could you tell her?

7.4   Catalogue Offer

ELISA

ELISA means enzyme-linked immunosorbent assay. It is a procedure which proves the existence of antibodies by enzymatic colour reactions. But also proteins, viruses, hormones, pesticides as well as toxins can be proved.

ELISA Kits

PromoKine offers a range of highly specific and sensitive ELISA kits that meet the highest quality standards. They can be used for reliable and reproducible detection and quantitation of numerous biomolecules in cell biology research. The 96 assay plate can either be used at once or a desired number of assays can be used because the wells in the assay plates can be detached.

In addition, we offer ELISA Development Kits which are very economical in medium- to high-throughput application. The kits are intended for experienced ELISA users and contain all required reagents to assay your target protein/peptide in ten 96-well microtiter plates (approximately 1,000 assays).

We continuously add new ELISA kits to our inventory. For an up-to-date product list please visit www.promokine.info/ELISAs.

Cell Signalling: Cytokines, Growth Factors, Receptors and Ligands

Product	Product Description	Size	Catalog N°
4-1BB/CD137 ELISA Kit, human	Human soluble CD137 ($-1BB) ELISA	96 tests	PK-EL -66556
90K (Mac-2BP) ELISA Kit, human	Human Macrophage Galactose-Specific Lectin Binding Protein ELISA	96 tests	PK-EL- 69196

Exercise

Imagine you are a representative of Promokine and you should write an offer for a biotechnological company. Make yourself familiar with ELISA kits regarding quality, function and prices. Write also an answer to the offer.

Use the following notes to write an offer.

- Vielen Dank für die Anfrage
- Rabatt von 5 % bei einer Zahlung innerhalb 15 Tagen möglich
- Die Installation und Einführung des Geräts inbegriffen

- Wartung ebenso und erfolgt auf Anfrage
- Garantie für 5 Jahre
- Die Lieferung erfolgt frei Haus innerhalb zwei Wochen
- Gerne sind wir bereit auch andere Produkte vorzuführen
- Wir freuen wieder von Ihnen zu hören
- Mit freundlichen Grüßen
- Anlage: Angebot

Vocabulary:
Frei Haus: free domicile

7.5   Product Description

SIFIN Kligler-Eisen-Agar (KIA)
Kligler-Eisen-Agar (KIA)
(Eisen-Zweizucker-Agar nach Kligler)
Kligler IRON Agar (KIA)
(Double Sugar Iron Agar acc. to Klinger)
500 g
REF TN 1146
LOT 0530210
2014-02

Directions
Suspend 49.6 g in 1 litre of distilled water and heat until completely dissolved. Distribute into tubes and sterilise by autoclaving at 121 °C for 15 minutes. Allow to set as **slant** agar in slanted positions with equal length of **butt** and slant.

Directions for Preparing Kligler Urea Agar acc. to Bader and Hotz
Suspend 49.6 g in 1 litre distilled water and heat until completely dissolved. Autoclave at 121 °C for 15 minutes and cool down to 45–50 °C. Add 1 bottle of Urea Solution 40 % (REF TN 1308) per litre of culture medium (final urea concentration: 2 %). Mix well and fill into sterile tubes. Allow to set as slant agar with approximately equal/length of butt and slant.

Storage
Dry, tightly closed, at 10 … 25 °C.

Exercises
1. Translate the product description.
2. Explain the use of agar in detail.
   Vocabulary:
   butt – Hochschicht
   slant – Schrägschicht

7.6   Important Vocabulary in the Field of Manuals

Noun	Verb	Adjective
instruction manual – Bedienungsanleitung	to pour sth. off – etw. abgießen	energised – unter Spannung stehen
instruction for use – Gebrauchsanweisung	to discard – abschalten	appropriate – sachgemäß
test records – Versuchsbeschreibung	to service sth. – etw. warten	thorough – sorgfältig
startup – Inbetriebnahme	to execute sth. – etw. durchführen	accessible – zugänglich
device – Gerät	to label sth. – etw. beschriften	impeccable – einwandfrei
lids – Deckel	to remove sth. – etw. entfernen	adjustable – justierbar
leads – Kabel	to proceed – weiter machen	explicit – deutlich
runtime – Laufzeit	to pipet/to pipette – pipettieren	hereditary – Erb-
power cable – Netzkabel	to spin – drehen	required – erforderlich
guarantee – Garantie	to observe the rules – die Vorschriften einhalten	maintained – gewartet

Bibliography

Instruction Manual
www.riele.de
Bedienungsanleitung Photometer 5010vs+
Robert Riele GmbH & CoKG
Kurfürstenstr. 75–79
13467 Berlin

Software Version 7.2
Dokumentation Ausgabe 08.2018

Test Records
www.bio-rad.com

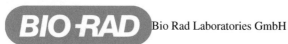 Bio Rad Laboratories GmbH

Kapellenstr. 12
85622 Feldkirchen

Biotechnology Explorer™
Chromosome 16:
PV92 PCR Informatics Kit
Catalog#166-2100EDU
Explorer.bio-rad.com

Instruction for Use
www.hermle-labortechnik.de
Hermle Labortechnik, Bedienungsanleitung für Mini Zentrifuge Z 130 M
Siemensstr. 25
78564 Wehingen

Catalogue Offer

www.promokine.info/ELISAs
Cell biology products – 2011/2012
PromoCell GmbH
Sickingerstr. 63/65
69125 Heidelberg

Product Description

www.sifin.de
SIFIN diagnostics GmbH Institut für Immunpräparate und Nährmedien GmbH Berlin
Berliner Allee 317–321
13088 Berlin

Presentation of a BIOTA's Work

8

Contents

The chapter should give the BIOTAs the occasion to enrich their vocabulary about their work, to present their practical training and to analyse job offers.

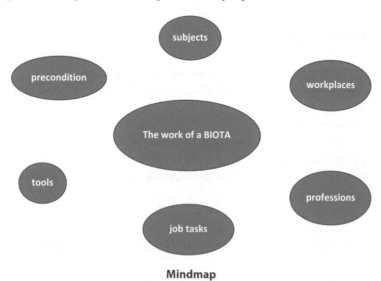

Mindmap

© Springer-Verlag GmbH Deutschland, ein Teil von Springer Nature 2020
U. Steiner, *Fachenglisch für BioTAs und BTAs*,
https://doi.org/10.1007/978-3-662-60666-7_8

8.1   Complete the Mindmap with at Least 5 Words

E.g.: precondition: O-level
subjects: biotechnology
workplaces: laboratory in companies and at universities
tools: photometer
job tasks: analyse DNA
professions: head of laboratory

8.2   Write a Coherent Text About the Work of a BIOTA with the Following Topics

Clarify the preconditions to become a BIOTA.
Elucidate professions related to a BIOTA.
Research chances of promotion for BIOTAs.
Find out the specific subjects which are taught for BIOTAs.
Explain job tasks related to specific biotechnological tools.
State some workplaces for BIOTAs.
Which field would you like to work in as a BIOTA.
Give reasons for your statement!
Summarise the advantages and disadvantages in the job of a BIOTA.
Draw a conclusion!

8.3   Job Offers for BIOTAs

1. Do research about job offers for BIOTAs. State some examples.
2. If you could choose your future workplace, describe what are the "must haves" of your future job?
3. State the structure of a job offer.
4. Write an answer for a job offer of a BIOTA in English!
   Make up your mind concerning the criteria of a letter of application.
5. In English speaking countries video interviews are very common as a job interview! What do you think about that?

8.4   Presentation About Your Four Weeks Practical Training

The following points have to be included in your presentation:

1. Presentation on foil or via power point with the following topics and a clearly arranged outline:

   A Short description about the company

   Special fields of the company

   Number of employees

   Structure of the company

   B Activity during the practical training

   C Detailed explanation of unknown vocabulary – extra list

   D Own short conclusion – positive and negative conclusion

2. Valuation criteria:

   10 points for the contents

   (complete presentation of the above mentioned points)

   10 points for the kind of presentation

   (clear structure, variety, optic presentation, self presentation)

   10 points for the language

   (fluency, free talk, understandability, error rate)

Small Talk in the Laboratory

9

Contents

Small talk is a way to open doors for future networks, for showing good intercultural manners and also being able to do marketing for your company. One should not underestimate the art of small talk.

Several exercises such as listening comprehension, inventing your own dialogue should strengthen your oral practice.

9.1 General Questions

1. Can you state the persons involved in the small talk.
2. Elucidate the usage of small talk in the laboratory.
3. Explain the aim of small talk.
4. State at least five typical small talk sentences!
5. Give a structure of a small talk conversation!
6. Complete the bubbles below!
7. Write your own small talk conversation with your partner!

Elektronisches Zusatzmaterial Die elektronische Version dieses Kapitels enthält Zusatzmaterial, das berechtigten Benutzern zur Verfügung steht (https://doi.org/10.1007/978-3-662-60666-7_9).

© Springer-Verlag GmbH Deutschland, ein Teil von Springer Nature 2020   147
U. Steiner, *Fachenglisch für BioTAs und BTAs*,
https://doi.org/10.1007/978-3-662-60666-7_9

9.2   Listening Comprehension

1. **Fill in the missing words:**
   I would like to _____ Mrs. Martin.
   She _____ for 20 years _____.
   May I _____ around. Please do not _____ to ask questions.
2. **Right or wrong**: (If the answer is wrong, correct it).
   A – The purpose of the visit is a common research project.
   _____

   B – They agreed upon a further visit in GB.
   _____

   C – Mrs. Martin gave detailed information about their company.
   _____

3. **Questions**:
   1. Describe the use of small talk.
   2. Summarise the whole conversation!
   3. Explain the usage of networks for biotechnological companies.

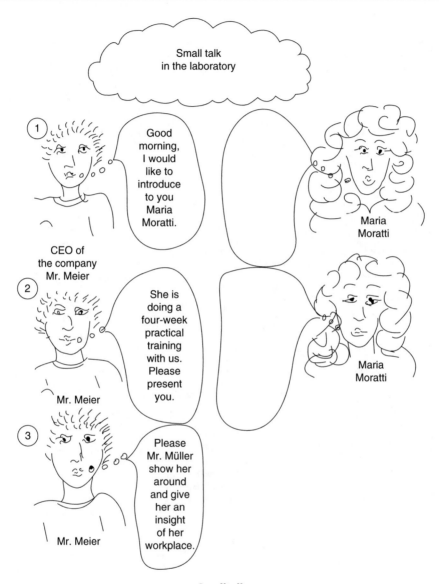

Smalltalk

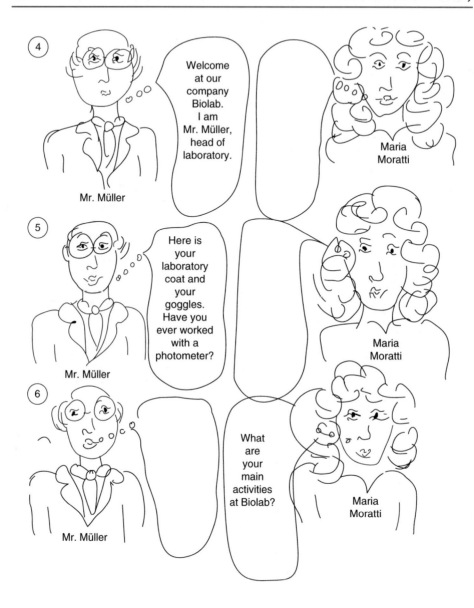

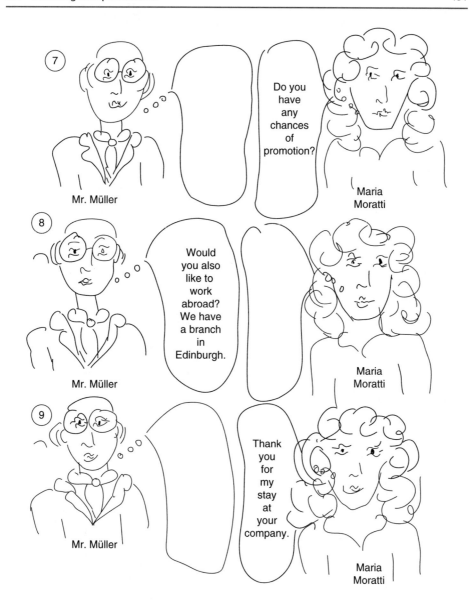

Further Education for BIOTAS

10

Contents

As biotechnology is in a steady changing progress, BIOTAs have to keep up with the cutting-edge processes. Therefore further education is an important topic.

10.1   Explain the Importance of Further Education

Find at least 10 reasons:

1. _____
2. _____
3. _____
4. _____
5. _____
6. _____
7. _____
8. _____
9. _____
10. _____

© Springer-Verlag GmbH Deutschland, ein Teil von Springer Nature 2020   153
U. Steiner, *Fachenglisch für BioTAs und BTAs*,
https://doi.org/10.1007/978-3-662-60666-7_10

10.2   Choose One Further Education Out of These Three Examples

Give at least ten reasons why you have chosen the further education. Write a coherent text!

Further Education 1: Biosciences
Process development for the purification of biopharmaceuticals
   Introduction to downstream Processing

Date: 3rd to 4th June, 20XX
Location: Frankfurt am Main
Head: Prof. Dr. Sonja Berensmeier
Fees: Member Euro 880,-
             Non-members Euro 960,-

Biopharmaceuticals as well as antibodies and therapeutic enzymes have to fulfill a very high purity and certain quality requirements after their biotechnological production and for further applications. It is the aim to give a fast insight of the basic knowledge of the process development, the downstream processing and every singular central procedure step on a technical scale.

Further Education 2
Summer Program Food Product Development at Sup'Biotech: 2019
   Introduction
Sup'Biotech is a private engineering school located in the Paris metropolitan area that is specialized in various emerging biotechnology-related fields. Sup'Biotech is part of the IONIS Institute of Technology cluster.

It is one of the top biotech schools in France and is part of IONIS, France's leading higher private education group. Its students go on into top positions in an array of industries including the health, bioinformatics, pharmaceutical and cosmetics industries, green industries and agribusiness.

Presentation
Sup'Biotech's unique curriculum combines science and engineering coursework with management skills and industry-specific technical knowledge, preparing students for dynamic careers in research, management, and communication roles. Our graduates possess not only the expertise needed in STEM-based careers but the interpersonal and management skills to effectively deliver their message.

The summer program Food Product Development takes place on our campus from July 1st to July 20th. Students come from around the world to study in English, go on our cultural trips and befriend other students from different cultures in an experience often described by participants as "unforgettable." Our students also learn about the domestic and international biotechnology markets. Sup'Biotech's professors come from diverse training and educational backgrounds such as universities, research centers, and industry.

Sup'Biotech's students are prepared for a wide range of responsibilities in various biotechnology and international corporations, working in the fields of health, cosmetics, the environment, pharmaceuticals and agribusiness.

Food Product Development

New food products are developed and tested every day, then brought to market by companies that have spent millions on R&D. This program has been designed to help our students intimately understand this process. Students will perform food science-related lab work and develop food products, culminating in a project that combines product design with business and marketing concepts. Lab work is coupled with market research and business implementation to give students a realistic look at the food science industries.

Who can apply to Sup'Biotech Summer School?

Applicants must have completed at least 2 years of studies in Life Sciences or Applied Sciences.

Programs are taught in English students must justify English language skills Language requirements CECRL B2 – IELTS 5,5/6 – TOEIC 600 – TOEFL IBT 65. Students can also provide a certificate or attestation from their home university demonstrating their knowledge of English. The number of participants is limited. Make sure to register early.

When?

July 1st–July 20th, 202X

Deadlines

Application deadline: May 30th, 202X

Payment deadline: May 31st, 202X

How to apply?

To complete your application, you will need to download the following documents:

Copy of Passport

CV in English

Last two transcripts

English Certificate (if required)

Cultural trips and site visits

The Summer Program is as much about having fun as it is about learning! During the program, students make the most of their time in France by going on a boat tour down the Seine River, visiting a huge indoor waterpark, going to an action adventure park called Koezio, visiting the Palace of Versailles and spending a day at Disneyland Paris, among other trips. They also visit biotech conferences, a brewery and other trips designed to show the application side of biotechnology.

Language courses

Included in the program fees are language courses. "Survival French" will be given to students who need to brush up their French skills. Students who already speak French fluently will be given "Scientific English" classes that give a new level of refinement to their spoken and technical English (2 ECTS credits for language).

Price

Application fees: 60 Euro

Program fees: 2350 Euro

Courses, including room, breakfast and lunch on weekdays, Language courses (French or English) biotech visits, all cultural activities and trips, the farewell party, a 3-week Paris transport pass and a lot more! You will receive a lab coat emblazoned with Sup'Biotech's logo.

If you are a student of one of Sup'Biotech's Partner institutions, please contact us: a special discount will apply!

Options: – Shuttle service: 100 Euro. If you take this optional charge, a shuttle service will pick you up from the airport and take you to your home in Paris and back to the airport at the end of the program, the price may vary.

Housing

Students live in shared rooms in Paris with host families or in Student apartments (with full access to a kitchen). Sup'Biotech has worked with host families extensively; they ensure students have an insight into French culture and are well-provided for.

Students will receive a certificate granting them the equivalent of 6 ECTS

Language: 2 ECTS

Seminars, courses: 2 ECTS

Projects: 2 ECTS

Program taught in:

English

Further Education 3: Biotechnology and Genetics
(Offered by Oxford Summer Courses)

Learning

Outline

How does biotechnology and genetics affect our everyday lives?

Find out on our thought-provoking course. Study Biotechnology and Genetics with us and you'll widen your skills and build your grasp on one of the most significant areas of science in the modern world. Study solo and collaborate with some of the finest academic minds. You'll trace research back through the ages to the present day to explore genetic engineering feats and what the future holds.

Teaching methodology

Learn the Oxford way with tutorial style teaching. Your expert tutor will foster self-directed learning and critical thinking through interactive seminars in small groups (no bigger than 8). During your course, you will complete two pieces of independent work (essays or problem sheets), which your tutor will then evaluate in either 1:1 or 2:1 tutorial. Tutorials will provide with the opportunity to discuss your work and feedback with your tutor and learn new perspectives from your classmates. On competition of the course, you'll receive a certificate and letter of recommendation from your tutor.

The Experience

It's all about balance. Study with us at Cambridge and we'll help you embrace everything the city has to offer – from socializing with new friends with shared interests to field trips and excursions for practical lessons you just can't learn from a textbook. We understand students. We make sure you are stimulated with a social calendar that packs it all in, from traditional guided tours of the University museums to a tranquil afternoon punting on the River Cam.

And of course, you'll experience the true Cambridge way of life from weekly formal dinners to competitive debating and croquet. Remember to save some energy for dancing the night away at a disco!

Stay in Cambridge

Home to Cambridge University since 1209, this city is famous for its cyclists, its museums, and of course, the 107 Nobel Laureates. But have you heard of the Mathematical Bridge (c. 1749). The first bridge built using mathematical principles? Or did you know that the first official game of football with rules similar to those we use now was played in 1848 in the middle of the city? Cambridge has so much to offer, from a vibrant history to cobbled streets and cozy cafes. It's the perfect place to study, and spend a summer exploring.

Date: June/July

Room type: Standard or Twin, shared bathroom

Price: 4848 Pounds

(as of October 20XX. For full details visit www.oxfordsummercourses.com)

10.3   What Are Quality Criteria for Good Further Education?

State at least five:

1. _____
2. _____
3. _____
4. _____
5. _____

Bibliography

Further Education 1
www.gdch.de/fortbildung

Further Education 2
www.supbiotech.fr

Further Education 3
www.oxfordsummercourses.com

Working with Specific Dictionaries

11

Contents

Nowadays everybody looks something quickly up in the internet without understanding the context or going into the great number of details you can use an online dictionary for. This chapter should make people aware of thoroughly choosing the right word in the right context with correct spelling.

11.1 General Questions

1. State ten criteria which you can look up in a dictionary.

1. _____   6. _____
2. _____   7. _____
3. _____   8. _____
4. _____   9. _____
5. _____   10. _____

© Springer-Verlag GmbH Deutschland, ein Teil von Springer Nature 2020
U. Steiner, *Fachenglisch für BioTAs und BTAs*,
https://doi.org/10.1007/978-3-662-60666-7_11

11.2   Compare Three Online Dictionaries!

What are their similarities? What are their differences?

	dictionary 1	dictionary 2	dictionary 3
criteria 1			
criteria 2			
criteria 3			
criteria 4			
criteria 5			
criteria 6			
criteria 7			
criteria 8			
criteria 9			
criteria 10			

1. Give reasons which online dictionary you think is the best one!
2. Find a definition for the following words:
   a. biotechnology
   b. antiputrefactive
   c. acetogenesis
   d. actual count

Apply the ten criteria of the table to the words 4a–d.

11.3   Partner Work: Pronunciation

See Figs. 11.1 and 11.2

Tandempartner A controls the partner B's pronounciation of the following words by listening to the online version of an online dictionary. Where is the stress of the word?

Sign for stress = '.

    1. determine

    2. pharmaceuticals

    3. biodegradable

    4. fungi

    5. constituents

Fig. 11.1 Tandempartner A

Tandempartner B control the partner A's pronounciation of the following words by listening to the online version of an online dictionary. Where is the stress of the word?

Sign for stress = '.

      1. mitochondrium

      2. vaccine

      3. supernatant

      4. eukaryote

      5. carcinogen

Fig. 11.2 Tandempartner B

Analysing Websites About Biotechnology

12

The essential knowledge about valuable and reliable good biotechnological websites should be made aware in this chapter by compiling good criteria for good websites.

Choose one website which deals with biotechnology. It should be a website of a company, an institution or an informative platform about biotechnology.

You should analyse and present this website regarding the outer appearance and the contents. Draw a conclusion. Would you recommend this website, if yes why, if no why?

E.g. how user-friendly is the website? Is the website well-structured and so on.

© Springer-Verlag GmbH Deutschland, ein Teil von Springer Nature 2020
U. Steiner, *Fachenglisch für BioTAs und BTAs*,
https://doi.org/10.1007/978-3-662-60666-7_12

Outer appearance and technical application:	Contents:
Criteria 1: e.g. user-friendliness	**Critera 1: contents of the menu**
Critera 2:	Criteria 2:
Critera 3:	Criteria 3:
Critera 4:	Criteria 4:
Critera 5:	Criteria 5:
Critera 6:	Criteria 6:
Critera 7:	Criteria 7:
Critera 8:	Criteria 8:
Critera 9:	Criteria 9:
Critera 10:	Criteria 10:

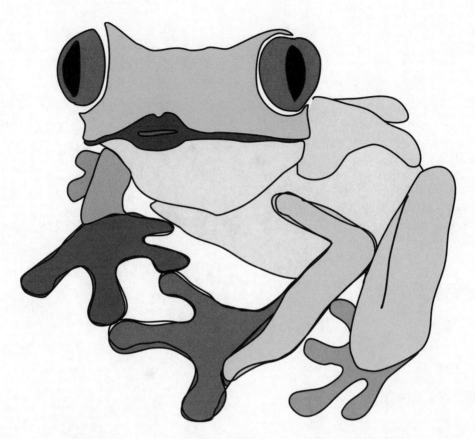

Erratum zu: Fachenglisch für BioTAs und BTAs

Erratum zu:
U. Steiner, *Fachenglisch für BioTAs und BTAs*,
https://doi.org/10.1007/978-3-662-60666-7_13

Der auf S. 82 fälschlicherweise gesetzte Kommentar der Autorin „Habe ich Ihnen geschickt / Das arabische Wort für Chemie kommt hier rein" wurde entfernt.

Die Zeilenangaben in den Vokabeltabellen auf S. 12, 22, 29 und 41 wurden entfernt.

Die aktualisierte Version dieses Buches finden Sie unter
https://doi.org/10.1007/978-3-662-60666-7_1
https://doi.org/10.1007/978-3-662-60666-7_2
https://doi.org/10.1007/978-3-662-60666-7_3
https://doi.org/10.1007/978-3-662-60666-7_4
https://doi.org/10.1007/978-3-662-60666-7_5
https://doi.org/10.1007/978-3-662-60666-7_7

© Springer-Verlag GmbH Deutschland, ein Teil von Springer Nature 2020
U. Steiner, *Fachenglisch für BioTAs und BTAs*,
https://doi.org/10.1007/978-3-662-60666-7_13

Printed in the United States
By Bookmasters